MEDITERRANEAN DIET PLAN:

The First Complete Guide

Mediterranean Diet, Cookbook and Healthy Recipes for Burn Fat, Plant, Reset your Metabolism and Weight Loss,

4-Week Mediterranean diet Plan,

Mindset Paradox for Success

Table of Contents

Introduction 1
Chapter 1: Why the Mediterranean Diet? 3
Chapter 2: Mindset for Your Diet Success 9
Chapter 3: Basic Principles.. 15
Chapter 4: Exercise Is Essential 29
Chapter 5: 4-Week Meal Plan... 33
Chapter 6: Recipes for the Summer 44
Chapter 7: Recipes for the Fall & Autumn Months 76
Chapter 8: Recipes for the Winter Months 107
Chapter 9: Recipes for the Spring Months 140
Conclusion 175
Index for the Recipes 176

Introduction

Congratulations on downloading the *MEDITERRANEAN DIET PLAN: The First Complete Guide Mediterranean Diet, Cookbook And Recipes, Plan, Guide With Exercise For Weight Loss, 4-Week Mediterranean Diet Plan, Mindset Paradox For Success*. Thank you for doing so. I am so excited that you have chosen to take a new path using the Mediterranean way of eating. Before we proceed, here's a bit of history.

Ancel Keys, a scientist, and his colleagues including Paul Dudley which later became President Eisenhower's cardiac physician conducted a *Seven Countries Study* in the years following World War II. The study compared individuals in the United States to those living in Crete - a Mediterranean island. Keys examined the plan testing people of all ages using the Mediterranean Diet.

The study examined 13,000 middle-aged men in Finland, the United States, the Netherlands, Yugoslavia, Greece, Italy, and Japan. It became evident the fruits, vegetables, grains, beans, and fish were the healthiest meals possible - even after the impoverishment of WWII. All of these discoveries were just the starting point.

Many benefits will be discussed including how you can lose and maintain a healthy weight in a sustainable way. Each chapter will carry you through different aspects of the plan and how you can go about changing your eating patterns with the Mediterranean diet.

You will also discover while on the Mediterranean diet plan, you will have more energy, and with that energy, you can become more active. Motivation will be the leader as you head toward your new lifestyle making essential changes along the path to success. Now it's time to learn how to use the techniques of the Mediterranean Diet Plan.

After you have the basics, you will enjoy a 28-day menu plan with all of the recipes included. Let's Get Started!

Chapter 1: Why the Mediterranean Diet?

The Mediterranean way of eating is typically rich in healthy plant foods and lower in animal foods. It places more of a focus on fish and seafood. It is predominantly beneficial because, at the end of the day, you won't be hungry!

The Mediterranean diet emphasizes that you get plenty of exercises, and primarily consume foods such as fruits, vegetables, legumes and nuts, and whole grains. You should consider replacing butter with healthier fats including canola or olive oil. Instead of salt, use spices and different herbs. Stick by the Mediterranean pyramid of foods and you won't go wrong!

Enjoy meals with family and friends using your new-found recipes and methods. Enjoy poultry and fish at least twice a week and have an occasional glass of red wine.

Health Benefits

The Mediterranean Plan is built upon healthy fats as well as plant-based foods.
Since the plan does not eliminate entire food groups, it is believed you should not have any problems complying with it in the long term.

You will have a lowered risk of strokes and heart disease. Patients who use the plan have had lowered level of oxidized low-density lipoprotein or LDL cholesterol. This is the bad cholesterol that can build up in your arteries.

The Mediterranean diet is rich in alpha-linolenic acid which is found in extra-virgin olive oil. The Warwick Medical School involved participants in a study who consumed more EVOO versus sunflower oil. The olive oil totals were much higher for decreased blood pressure. Lowered hypertension is another benefit achieved by consuming olive oil because it helps keep the arteries clear and dilated. It makes the nitric oxide more bioavailable. The healthy fats also make you less likely to struggle to maintain cholesterol levels.

Strokes can be caused by bleeding in the brain or a blocked blood vessel. You may notice numbness, weakness, headaches, confusion, vision problems dizziness, or slurred speech. The diet helps with these issues.

Your vision will improve. You might be able to stave off - or even prevent the risk of macular degeneration which is the major cause for adults over 54 losing their eyesight. The condition affects over ten million Americans and can destroy the area of your retina which is responsible for clear vision. The vegetables and fish with the omega-3 fatty acids are the providers to lower or reduce the risk entirely. Also, you will have less chance of having cataracts with the consumption of green leafy veggies which have lutein.

You will drop the pounds using healthier practices. Your search is over if you are seeking a plan that is worthwhile. The Med Plan, as it is sometimes called, has been proven to work for weight loss easily and naturally with its many nutrient-dense foods. The focus is placed on healthy fats to keep the carbs moderately low and improve high-quality proteins. The healthy fats, protein, and fiber keep you much more satisfied than candy, chips, or cookies. The veggies make up the bulk of the meal by filling your stomach, so you don't feel hungry an hour after your meal, and you won't receive a spike your blood sugar.

You will experience improved agility. Studies have shown up to 70% of the seniors who are at risk of developing frailty or other muscle weaknesses have reduced the risks factors using the plan.

You will enjoy eating natural foods. The Mediterranean diet is low in sugar and processed foods. You can certainly appreciate a diet or a way of life that is close to nature, especially if you can locate some locally produced organic sources. People in the Mediterranean enjoy the same types of delicious desserts and many are made using natural sweeteners such as honey.

Improved asthma symptoms are evident from those using the plan. Numerous studies have revealed the antioxidant diet helped children who followed the plan emphasizing the intake of plant-based foods and lower intake of red meats.

Risk factors for Alzheimer's are reduced. Research has deemed a 40% reduction occurs for those who use the diet plan, and the risk factors associated with Alzheimer's. Dementia may progress in the later stages of Alzheimer's which can be treated with medication and aided by the Mediterranean plan. You should also consider some additional exercise to slow the process.

Reduction in Parkinson's risk factors has been observed. The risk of the disease is cut in half because the high levels of antioxidants in the diet prevent oxidative stress, which is the cell-damaging process. Parkinson's disease affects the cells in your brain which produce dopamine. You may have some issues with gait and speech patterns, tremors, and muscle rigidity issues. The Mediterranean diet can help safeguard you from Alzheimer's which are triggered by thinking, judgment, and memory losses.

The Mediterranean Plan has helped those with diabetes. The Mediterranean Diet controls excessive insulin which is a hormone that controls your blood sugar levels and can cause you to gain weight and keep it on, no matter what you do to try to lose it. The well-balanced diet which is low in sugar and contains healthy fatty acids can create a balance so your body can burn off the fat and give you more energy at the same time.

The diet is considered lower in saturated fat, but higher in fat than the American standard diet plans, according to the *American Heart Association*. The combination is usually 20-30% quality protein foods, 30-40% healthy fats, and 40% complex carbs. This creates the balance to keep your hunger under control and the weight gain down which is an excellent way to keep insulin levels normalized.

As a result, with the energy levels up, so should your mood. Sugar is usually consumed through dessert, fruit, or wine. The balance also prevents the 'highs and lows' which is the mood- altering factor. Most individuals on the plan will eat a balanced breakfast within one or two hours from the time the day starts, which is the time of day the lowest levels of blood sugar are present in the healthy fats and fibers, along with three meals each day to maintain the balance.

The Delicious Path to Weight Loss

You can plan healthy choices for breakfast, lunch, and dinner, but what about your snacking habits? You should choose a healthy snack which would be around the 150-200 calorie marker. Choose a grapefruit, apple, or pear. Add a pinch (⅛ of a teaspoon) of sea salt for a change. This treat will help fend off the hunger cravings. You want it to contain some whole-grain sources, some carbs, and protein to promote satiety.

The path to weight loss is the best way to lose weight using healthy food choices. These are just a few examples of some of the foods you can enjoy when you just do not have the time for a meal:

Nut Butter & Fruit Slices: Pears and apples are a hit when you prepare your favorite nut butter. Cashew butter and almond butter are two healthy choices that contain heart-healthy fats. By roasting and blending the raw almonds, you are ensured to receive all of the rich fiber, protein, and fats that your body needs to remain active.

Dates & Figs: These are some products which grow well in the Mediterranean climate. They are also a sweet treat when you are too busy to prepare a snack.

Tuna Salad & Crackers: It is time to move away from the traditional tuna salad. Substitute oil-packed tuna with a splash of red vinegar wine, scallions, and a squeeze of mustard. Add some whole wheat crackers for a mid-morning treat.

Greek Yogurt & Fruit: Enjoy a protein-rich snack of some Greek yogurt. Garnish the yogurt with some sunflower seeds, a handful of berries, and a drizzle of honey for a tasty mid-afternoon snack.

Sun-Dried Tomato & Goat Cheese Spread: The rich flavor of the sun-dried tomatoes are only the beginning since it is full of calcium, iron, vitamin C, vitamin A, and lycopene. It also provides a heart-healthy boost since it is often packed in olive oil. Smear a layer of goat cheese on whole wheat crackers and top it off with some sun-dried tomatoes for a quick snack. Add a snip of basil on top of each cracker for a few additional vitamins and minerals.

Kalamata Olives: When you are in a rush, nothing says it all like a handful of healthy olives. They are rich in many antioxidants including oleic acid, tyrosol, and hydroxytyrosol. Mix them up with a small amount of feta cheese for an additional boost.

Pita & Hummus: You can have some sesame paste (tahini) and chickpeas in the form of hummus. Consider making some at home, but you can also purchase it ready-made. Make sure you read the label and choose one with a limited amount of preservatives. You can choose a whole-wheat piece of pita bread with a hummus spread for a delicious snack.

Chapter 2: Mindset for Your Diet Success

Research has proven time and again that you have to get in the right mindset to drop the unwanted pounds. Shifting your mindset is about how to lose weight from the outside without realizing the intention. Don't expect quick fixes. All it takes is willpower and setting realistic goals to be successful during your journey through the Mediterranean diet weight loss plan.

If you are choosing to drop the pounds and keep them off, you will discover the Mediterranean style is the cure you have been seeking. You have to get motivated to get any plan to work for you. The first step was taken since you purchased this informative guide.

Jot down your goals and the reasons you need to change your eating patterns. As you proceed with your weight loss, keep your motivation in check by referring to those reasons. It will give you a needed boost.

Surround yourself with people that are positive; you will develop emotionally healthy realistic goals. Dropping the pounds will be the result, but first, you need to set goals. You need to make the goals small with sustainable things that you have full control over to be successful. You can make simple goals such as how many servings of fruits you will eat in one day or how many hours of sleep you will have that night.

It is essential for you to recharge and take the evening hours to relax and improve your sleep hygiene. Try to leave work – at work. Deal with the issues when you return. If you are going through a tough time or working long hours, you tend to forget items you may 'munch' on as you are working. Make it a point to write down everything you eat.
Working long hours can be beneficial for knocking off those pounds, but it can also cause you to be restless and can lead to post-workout insomnia if you have worked out or done other strenuous physical activities on your evenings off.

No matter what the case, slow down for at least an hour or more before attempting to retire for the evening.

If you have dieted before, you already know you will reach spans of time where your weight loss will level out. That's merely a segment of weight loss that can't be moderated. All you need to do is remain consistent. The weight loss will return. It is much better to expect problems or roadblocks than it is to believe that the new dieting methods will be smooth sailing.

Set a timeline with realistic goals. Choosing to lose weight is a fantastic move, but you need to be realistic. You might find it helpful to use baby steps to achieve the desired goal. For example, set a goal to lose six pounds in the next five to six weeks when you begin your new Mediterranean diet plan. For most people, healthy benefits are received if you start the plan by losing five to ten percent of your starting weight. It may not be your ideal medically suggested weight, but it is going to lead you toward a healthier weight. Take baby steps.

Consider what you want to change about the way you feel concerning your weight issues. If you notice you are craving sweets, your plan should include a way to reduce your intake down to two times weekly. Provide you and your family with healthier, filling choices such as fruit. However, don't go cold turkey because the plan won't work. Search for a recipe that allows you to taste the sweetness without the additional calories.

After you have adjusted your body to the Mediterranean way of eating, be willing to change your goals as you make progress. By starting small, you leave the door open so you can make more significant challenges as you proceed through the plan.

Make Healthier Food Choices: Make Substitutions:

- **Breadcrumbs**: You can still enjoy your crunchiness by replacing regular breadcrumbs with crushed pork rinds. The good news is that the pork rinds have zero carbs. Next time, enjoy healthier fats.

- **Pasta**: Replace pasta using zucchini. Use a spiralizer and make long ribbons to cover your plate. It is excellent for many dishes served this way.
  For example, you can also prepare spaghetti squash for regular spaghetti.

- **Tortillas**: Get ready to say no to this one which weighs in at approximately 98 grams for just 1 serving. Instead, enjoy a lettuce leaf at about 1 gram per serving. You will still have a healthy crunch to enjoy!

Portion Control

You need to be aware of the foods you are consuming. This takes good management skills. It is important to set guidelines while on the Mediterranean diet plan. You need to gauge each portion of the food that you're eating to ensure you're getting the correct calorie intake daily. The following lists are just a few examples of how you would portion their foods during your dieting journey:

- *Vegetables*: One cup of raw leafy veggies or one-half cup of all others

- *Fruit*: One orange, one apple, one banana, 30 grams: 1.1 ounces of grapes: 7.1 ounces of watermelon or other melons

- *Legumes*: 100 grams (One cup) of dry cooked beans

- *Grains*: 50 to 60 grams (.5 cup) of cooked pasta or rice: One slice of bread is 25 grams (almost an ounce)
- *Dairy*: One cup of yogurt or one cup of milk, 30 grams, or about 1.1 ounces of cheese or 1 egg.
- *Meat*: 60 grams (2.1 ounces) of fish or lean meat
- *Potatoes*: 100 grams (3.5 ounces)
- *Nuts*: 30 grams (1.1 ounces) Sprinkled on foods for flavor or as a snack

With the right combination of foods, you can set and keep your goals.

Imagine Your Future:

I always try to plan for the future since no one is promised tomorrow. The Mediterranean diet will meet your needs because it is a very sustainable diet plan.

Think about it, this book of guidelines will get you off to the right start with your prepared meal plan. All you have to do is take away the foods you don't like and replace them with Mediterranean diet foods that work. Just so you know how well the plan works, take a snapshot now and save it to your phone. After you have a month or so on the plan, take another snapshot and compare the two.

Consider using free apps to help you track your weight loss. You'll want to keep track of what you eat every day. Research has shown individuals who keep records of their food activity will more than likely be successful with weight loss. You will always be able to move forward when you discover any weaknesses that exist in your dieting success.

- MyFitnessPal has been chosen as one of the best apps available to track your macros. It's free to download, but you can also choose to update to a premium plan for higher rates.
- My Food Diary will provide you with the nutritional facts to ensure you have the correct carbohydrate, protein, and fats in your diet plan.

Prepare A Food Journal: If you cheat or go off of your scheduled meal plan, you should still add the additional calories into your daily log. It will be a reminder of your indulgence, but it will help keep you in line. All you need to do is update your journal regularly, and remain totally honest in the journal and write down all items.

By having a journal, you can document your food items from a different perspective on each day. Make comments over which foods you prepared, and whether you liked or disliked them.

You can also include your objectives of the plan; mention how you're doing on the diet, document your thoughts and feelings as well as your experience with others and yourself as you proceed through each week of the menu plan. Use patience and your time, and you'll appreciate the success you will be provided in the end.

Understand Your Cravings: If you have stood by your guideline and followed the plan, you should see a remarkable improvement. If not, don't give up; instead, just make adjustments and keep dieting.

Salty Foods: Your body is craving silicon. Have a few nuts and seeds; just be sure to count them into your daily counts.

Fatty or Oily Foods: The levels of calcium and chloride need repair with some spinach, broccoli, cheese, or fish.

Sugary Foods: Several things can trigger the desire for sugar, but typically phosphorous, and tryptophan are the culprits. Have some chicken, beef, lamb, liver, cheese, cauliflower, or broccoli.

Chocolate: The carbon, magnesium, and chromium levels are requesting a portion of spinach, nuts, and seeds, or some broccoli and cheese.

Chapter 3: Basic Principles

Learn How to Understand Nutrition Labels

Look for Short Ingredient List: The bulk of the food is listed in order according to weight and are usually the first ingredients. If you don't recognize an ingredient, place it back on the shelf! Consider using products that have no more than 5 ingredients. The longer ingredients probably are the result of unnecessary extras including artificial preservatives.

Check Serving Sizes: Packages often time contain more than a single serving. Visualize how many calories and the amount of sugar is in a single container. Thus, you need to check the serving size first.

Discover Calorie Counts: It is essential to check the labels calorie count since they are very important during your process using the Mediterranean diet plan.

Avoid Fats: It's important to remove foods from your diet plan that contain any fully hydrogenated or partially hydrogenated oils.

Check the Percent of Daily Value: The daily value will tell you how many nutrients are in each serving of a packaged item.

Get More Of These Nutrients: Look for calcium, iron, fiber, vitamin A, and vitamin C.

The Label Explained

- Serving Information At the Top: This provides the size of one serving and per container.
- Check the total calories per serving and container.
- Limit certain nutrients from your diet.
- Provide yourself with plenty of beneficial nutrients
- Understand the % of daily value section.

Avoid These Foods

- **Added Sugar:** Ice cream, candy, regular soda, plus many others.

- **Refined Oils**: Canola oil, cottonseed oil, soybean oil, etc.

- **Trans fats**: Found in various processed foods such as margarine, added sugar, ice cream, candies, table sugar, soda, and others. Added sugars, sugar-sweetened beverages, refined grains, processed meats, and other highly processed foods.

- **Processed Meat Products**: Hot dogs, processed sausages, bacon

- **Refined Grains**: Pasta made with refined wheat, white bread

Note If You Are Pregnant: You should avoid some of the oily fish such as swordfish, shark, and tuna because some may contain low levels of toxic heavy metals.

What to Eat Rarely:

- **Red meats** (Limit to once each week)

Foods You Can Eat

Seafood and Fish: Mussels, clams, crab, prawns, oysters, shrimp, tuna, mackerel, salmon, trout, sardines, anchovies, and more

Poultry: Turkey, duck, chicken, and more

Eggs: Duck, quail, and chicken eggs

Dairy Products: Contain calcium, B12, and Vitamin A: Greek yogurt, regular yogurt, cheese, plus others

Tubers: Yams, turnips, potatoes, sweet potatoes, etc.

Vegetables: Another excellent choice for fiber, and antioxidants: Cucumbers, carrots, Brussels sprouts, tomatoes, onions, broccoli, cauliflower, spinach, kale, eggplant, artichokes, fennel, etc.

Seeds and Nuts: Provide minerals, vitamins, fiber, and protein: Macadamia nuts, cashews, pumpkin seeds, sunflower seeds, hazelnuts, chestnuts, Brazil nuts, walnuts, almonds, pumpkin seeds, sesame, poppy, and more

Fruits: Excellent choices for vitamin C, antioxidants, and fiber: Peaches, bananas, apples, figs, dates, pears, oranges, strawberries, melons, grapes, etc.

Spices and Herbs: Cinnamon, garlic, pepper, nutmeg, rosemary, sage, mint, basil, parsley, etc.

Whole Grains: Whole grain bread and pasta, buckwheat, whole wheat, barley, corn, whole oats, rye, quinoa, bulgur, couscous

Legumes: Provide vitamins, fiber, carbohydrates, and protein: Chickpeas, pulses, beans, lentils, peanuts, peas

Healthy Fats: Avocado oil, avocados, and olives are excellent fats. The monounsaturated fat which is found in olive oil is a fat that can help reduce the 'bad' cholesterol. The oil has become the traditional fat worldwide with some of the healthiest populations. A great deal of research has been provided showing the oil is a huge plus towards the risk of heart disease because of the antioxidants and fatty acids.

You will still need to pay close attention when purchasing olive oil because it may have been extracted from the olives using chemicals or possibly diluted with other cheaper oils, such as canola and soybean. You need to be aware of refined or light olive or regular oils. The Mediterranean diet plan calls for the use of extra-virgin olive oil because it has been standardized for purity using natural methods providing the sensory qualities of its excellent taste and smell. The oil is high in phenolic antioxidants which makes—real—olive oil beneficial.

Beverage Options: Maintaining a healthy body requires plenty of water, and the Mediterranean diet plan is not any different. Tea and coffee are allowed, but you should avoid fruit juices or sugar-sweetened beverages that contain large amounts of sugar.

White Meats: White meats are high in minerals, protein, and vitamins but you should remove any visible fat and the skin.

Red Meats: You are allowed red meats including lamb, pork, and beef in small quantities. They are rich in minerals, vitamins, and protein—especially iron. Use caution because they do contain more fat—specifically saturated fat—compared to the fat content found in poultry. Don't leave it out entirely; save it for a special dinner or with a stew or casserole.

Potatoes: You have noticed that potatoes are listed in the tubers group because they are a healthy choice, but it will greatly depend on how they are prepared. You receive potassium, Vitamin B, Vitamin C, and some of your daily fiber nutrients. You must consider that they do contain large amounts of starch which can be quickly converted to glucose which can be harmful and place you at some risk of type 2 diabetes. Use simpler methods of cooking them including baking, boiling, and mashing them without butter.

Desserts and Sweets: Biscuits, cakes, and sweets should be consumed in small quantities, as a special treat. Not only is the sugar a temptation for type 2 diabetes; it can also promote tooth decay. Many times, they may also contain higher levels of saturated fats. You can receive some nutritional value, but as a general rule—stick to small portions.

What to Eat in Moderation: Eggs, poultry, milk, butter, yogurt, and cheese

Improve the Flavor of Foods

The use of her herbs and spices provide additional flavor and aroma to your foods while on the diet plan. It will also help reduce the need for salt or fat while you're preparing your meals. Spices and herbs which adhere to the standards of a traditional Mediterranean Diet include chiles, lavender, tarragon, savory, sumac, and zaatar.

These are a few more ways you can benefit from spices and herbs:

Anise Benefits: You can improve digestion as well as help reduce nausea and alleviate cramps. Prepare some anise tea after a meal to help treat indigestion and bloating gas as well as constipation.

Bay Leaf Benefits: Bay leaves contain magnesium, calcium, potassium, and Vitamins A & C. You are promoting your general health and it is also proven to be useful in the treatment of migraines.

Basil Benefits: You can receive aid in digestion, help with gastric diseases, and help reduce flatulence. You can also protect your heart health, help reduce stress and anxiety, and help manage your diabetes. The next time you have dandruff issues, try rubbing them in your scalp after shampooing. The chemicals help eliminate dandruff and dry skin.

Black Pepper Benefits: Pepper promotes nutrient absorption in the tissues all over your body, speeds up your metabolism, and improves digestion. The main ingredient of pepper is a pipeline which gives it the pungent taste. It can boost fat metabolism by as much as 8% for up to several hours after it's ingested. As you will see, it is used throughout your healthy Mediterranean recipes.

Cayenne Pepper Benefits: The secret ingredient in cayenne is the capsaicin which is a natural compound that gives the peppers the fiery heat. This provides a short increase in your metabolism. The peppers are also rich in vitamins, effective as an appetite controller, smoothes out digestion issues, and benefits your heart health.

Sweet & Spicy Cloves Benefits: Add cloves to hot tea for a spicy flavor. The antiseptic and germicidal ingredients in cloves will help with many types of pain including the relief of arthritis pain, gum and tooth pain, aids in digestive problems, and helps to fight infections. Use the oil of clove as an antiseptic to kill bacteria in fungal infections, itchy rashes, bruises, or burns. Just the smell of cloves can help encourage mental creativity.

Ground Chia Seeds Benefits: The seeds can absorb up to 11 times its weight in liquid. Be sure to add plenty of water and soak them for at least 5 minutes before using in your recipes. Otherwise, you will have some uncomfortable digestion after eating them. Be sure to remain hydrated.

Cumin Benefits: The flavor of cumin and has been described as spicy, earthy, nutty, and warm. It's been a long used as traditional medicine. It can help promote digestion and reduce foodborne infections. It is also beneficial for promoting weight loss and improving cholesterol and blood sugar control.

Fennel Benefits: You can receive potassium, sodium, vitamin A, calcium, vitamin C, iron, vitamin B6, and magnesium from fennel. Your bone health will show improvement with the phosphate and calcium which are excellent for your bone structure. Iron and zinc or crucial for the production of collagen. Your heart health is also protected with vitamin C, folate, potassium, and fiber provided in fennel.

Garlic Benefits: Garlic leads the charge on lowering your blood sugar and assisting you in weight loss. It helps control your appetite.

Ginger Benefits: Ginger is an effective diuretic which increases urine elimination. It is also known for his cholesterol-fighting properties, as a metabolism and mobility booster. Ginger also helps fight bloating issues.

Marjoram Benefits: This is used in the diet to promote healthy digestion, assist in the management of type 2 diabetes, helps to rectify hormonal imbalances, and also helps promote restful sleep and a sound mind.

Mint Benefits: Mint can be used for the treatment of nasal congestion, nausea, dizziness, and headaches. It helps to improve blood circulation, improves dental health, and helps colic in infants. Mint helps to prevent dandruff and pesky head lice.

Oregano Benefits: Oregano is very easily added to your diet and is rich in antioxidants and may also help fight bacteria. Oregano is also good for the treatment of the common cold since it helps in reducing infections, helps kill off intestinal parasites, and it's also beneficial in treating menstrual cramps. One huge plus is that it also supports the body with nutrients to help support weight loss and improve digestion.

Parsley Benefits: You can help your skin, prostate, and digestive tract by making use of its high levels of a flavonoid called apigenin. It contains a powerful antioxidant and inflammatory power as well as providing remarkable anti-cancer properties.

Rosemary Benefits: The spice is known to increase hair growth, may help relieve pain, eases stress, and also helps reduce joint inflammation.

Sage Benefits: The leaves of the sage plant are also used to make medicine. It is an excellent source to improve your digestive issues including diarrhea, stomach pain or gastritis, heartburn, and gas or flatulence. It is also beneficial for those who suffer from depression, Alzheimer's disease, memory loss, and so much more.

Tarragon Benefits: The tarragon spice is an excellent choice for maintaining your blood sugar levels, keeping your heart healthy, reduction of inflammation symptoms, improvement of digestive functions, improves central nervous system conditions, and supports healthier eyes.

Thyme Benefits: Thyme is another spice which has been used throughout history for protection from 'Black Death' as well as for embalming. (Not a pretty thought for dinner but interesting nonetheless.) It is also believed to have insecticidal and antibacterial properties. You can use it as an essential oil, as a dried herb or fresh.

As you will notice, the recipes included in your new menu plan have an extensive listing of spices. Not only do they improve your foods, but also they improve your health at the same time!

Keep to the Diet

No more worrying, you are good to 'go' on the Mediterranean diet - even when you're out. Most restaurants are a reasonable choice for you while you are participating in this diet plan. Ask the waiter or waitress to cook your food using extra-virgin olive oil (EVOO) instead of butter. Choose to have a house salad and extra veggies. Have some seafood or other types of fish for the main entree. Eat whole-grain bread.

One huge advantage of the Mediterranean diet is that you can be flexible. These are a few additional tips for dining out beginning with the appetizers, entrees, beverages, and lastly desserts. So, let's get started.

Have a healthy snack before you leave home: One of the easiest ways to remain on your Mediterranean diet while dining out is to take the edge off of your hunger. Enjoy a high-protein and low-calorie snack such as yogurt to help you feel full. It will help you from overeating.

Enjoy a huge glass of ice water before and during your meal. Eliminate the sugary sweet drinks. Water cannot be stressed enough while you are attempting to drop the pounds since it helps keep you hydrated and steers the hunger away.

Suggestions for the Appetizers: Remove the temptation and ask the waiter/waitress not to bring a bread-and-butter basket to the table. If you are hungry, you may be tempted to eat more than you should. Avoid fried appetizers. Stick with some steamed fish or shellfish, mixed salads, broth-based soups, or grilled veggies. Share your appetizer, so you will have a smaller portion.

Suggestions for the Entree Course: Choose from lean pork (center-cut or tenderloin), fish, poultry, or vegetarian choices. If you are bound for red meat—choose the leaner cuts such as flank, sirloin, filet mignon, or a tenderloin. You might also want to consider the beef will have a higher calorie and higher fat count. Ask for substitutes for mashed potatoes, macaroni salad, potato salad, coleslaw, or French fries. Instead, choose a side salad, steamed rice, baked potato, or steamed veggies.

Use caution with sauces. Ask if it is oil based, or if cream or butter in the sauce. Avoid sauces with cream, cheese, oil, or butter. Request that the sauces be served in a separate container, so you can add what is allowed. Use your fork to dip the sauce to limit the temptation of over-indulging.

Enjoy your meal and eat slowly. Ask to have the plate removed when you feel full. Eat only half of the portion or share it with a friend. You can always ask for a bag to go and enjoy the leftovers later. It will be an excellent lunch meal. You can also ask for half of the meal to be held in the kitchen until you are through with your meal. Once again, just remove the temptation!

Make Healthier Beverage Choices: Have a non-caloric beverage like tea, seltzer water, water, sugar-free or diet soda. Choose a splash or orange juice or cranberry juice in some seltzer water for a fizzy surprise.

Make Healthy Dessert Choices: Have a cup of coffee, cappuccino, or some herbal tea with a sugar substitute or no sugar with some skim milk. Order a dessert for everyone at the table to enjoy. Order some berries or mixed fruit.

Slow Down: Try eating slower and chewing your food more thoroughly. Put your utensils down between mouthfuls to help slow you down. It will also give you time for satiety to kick in.

Prevent yourself from going to all you can eat buffets. This is a nightmare for portion control. Don't tempt fate if you're just beginning your new diet program. Choose a smaller plate when you go to the buffet. You can also choose a normal size plate or fill it half full of veggies or salad.

Restaurant Options for the Mediterranean Diet Plan

These are just a few of the ways to enjoy your outing:

McDonald's: These are some of the healthy choices:

- Apple Dippers with a low-fat caramel dip or a yogurt parfait.
- Caesar Salad & Grilled Chicken
- Bacon Ranch Salad & Grilled Chicken

Subway: Choose a Subway Club Salad, Savory Turkey Breast Salad, or many others. You can choose any 6-inch sub with the following ingredients:
- Roast Beef
- Oven Roasted Chicken Breast
- Savory Turkey Breast
- Subway Club
- Savory Turkey Breast & Ham
- Ham
- Honey Mustard Ham
- Sweet Onion Chicken Teriyaki

Taco Bell: You can cut the fats in your food by 25% if you order any of these items using the Fresco style which will provide 350 calories or less and under ten grams of fat. These are just two of your choices:

- Beef Soft Taco: 160-200 calories
- Burrito Supreme for 390-420 calories. The Fresco burrito is 340-350 calories.

Pyramid of the Mediterranean Diet

Overall: Yes, Plenty of water is at the head of the list for every day!

Your Monthly Allowance:

- 4 Servings - Red meat

Your Weekly Allowance:

- **3 Servings**: Eggs - Potatoes - Sweets
- **3-4 Servings**: Nuts, Olives, Pulses
- **7-14 tbsp.**: Olive oil
- **4 Servings**: Legumes - Poultry
- **5-6 Servings**: Fish

Your Daily Allowance:

- **3 Servings**: Fruit - Dairy Products
- **6 Servings**: Vegetables
- **8 Servings**: Non-refined products and cereals (brown rice, whole grain bread, etc.)

Olive Oil: Acts as a major added lipid

Learn Portion Control

These are some general guidelines so you can better calculate the serving sizes for your meal planning needs:

- **Meat**: 2.1 ounces of fish or lean meat
- **Potatoes**: 3.5 ounces

- **Vegetables**: 1 cup of raw - leafy veggies or .5 cup of all others
- **Dairy**: 1 cup of yogurt or 1 cup of milk; 1.1 ounces of cheese
- **Eggs**: 1 egg
- **Grains:** .5 cup cooked rice or pasta; 1 slice of bread is almost 1 ounce
- **Nuts**: 30 grams (1.1 ounces): Sprinkled on foods for flavor or as a snack
- **Legumes**: 100 grams (1 cup) of dry cooked beans
- **Fruit**: 1 orange, 1 apple, 1 banana, 1 ounce of grapes, 7.1 ounces of watermelon or other melons
- **Wine**: 125 ml or about a 4.2-ounce glass of a regular strength red wine

Chapter 4: Exercise Is Essential

Your weight will depend on the amount of energy your body burns and how much energy you consume from beverage and food products. Before we begin, let's discuss a little about the science of how weight loss works. In short, if you consume more calories (more food) than your body can use; you add on the pounds. The excess or extra energy is converted to fat and is stored in your body. If the ratio of the number of calories that you ingest equals the amount your body is using; your weight will remain stable or unchanged.

However, if you consume fewer calories than your body can use; you will lose weight. It requires your body to 'tap into' the stored body fat to obtain the additional energy needed. In one pound of fat, you receive about 3,500 calories. If you lower the calories by eating better on the plan; you can cut the calories by about 500 calories daily which can result in one pound of weight loss weekly.

This is the beauty of the Mediterranean way of eating healthier; you don't want to drop the pounds too quickly, but you could with a new eating pattern. If you lose more than one kilogram or about 2.2 pounds; instead of losing the unwanted fat, you might be losing muscle tissue instead. In short, that's why you need to get more exercise and eat fewer calories.

How to Proceed

It is important to increase your physical activities for about thirty minutes each day as part of your new diet regimen. You can begin slowly with a walk, go for a swim, go for a bicycle ride, or go for a jog.

If you have any other risk factors such as smoking; maybe it is time to consider breaking the habit. Have your blood pressure frequently checked, so you know your diet plan is working for you.

Research has shown if you have a strict Mediterranean diet, and exercise regularly; you can keep your weight under control. With the filling menus you will be planning, you won't be hungry and end up with unwanted calories or inches around your waistline. After all, a sedentary lifestyle is a major contributing factor to obesity.

Begin & Maintain a Regular Exercise Program

You should consider exercising 30-60 minutes daily as an integral part of healthy living choices. Regular physical activity benefits your strength, mood, and balance. If you've been living a more sedentary lifestyle, it's vital for you to speak with your doctor about a safe exercise regimen. Make sure you start off slow. Progressively pick up the pace and regularity of your workouts.

Physicians suggest patients suffering from pressure issues should engage in dynamic, moderate-intensity, aerobic exercise for a minimum of 1/2 hour each day. You can enjoy jogging, walking, swimming, or cycling on five days each week. Start using a pedometer and set a new goal of activity using a base of 10,000 steps daily. Get started with a group of friends and walk or start a workout group.

Plan Walking With the Family. Start making Saturday morning your 'walk day' for the entire family. Take a Sunday walk instead of taking a Sunday drive. Walk instead of driving, whenever you can. After the evening meal, go for a walk with the family. Make it a daily habit.

Go out Of Your Way to Walk: If you take a bus, make an early stop, and walk part of the way. When you go shopping, park a few aisles further away, and take a walk. While you are window shopping, go for a brisk walk in the mall. If you have a choice of an elevator or the stairs; burn a few calories!

These are a few examples of how to *moderately* burn those extra calories:

- Housework - 60 min.
- Cycling - 6 min.
- Walking - 15 min.
- Running - 10 min.
- Swimming laps - 20 min.

Regular exercise can help strengthen your muscles and keep them flexible. One huge benefit is its ability to help improve your sense of well-being and control your weight. However, cardiac patients should avoid running and white training without getting professional advice.

Try a few of these moves:

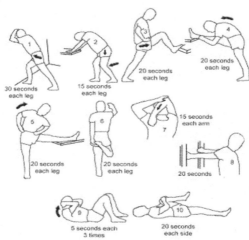

When you reach a goal, the important thing is to reward yourself.

Avoid distractions and relax. Leave the television off and take a leisurely a half-hour walk to remove the stress of the day. Just stay busy and your future will be much brighter with a much healthier outlook.

Chapter 5: 4-Week Meal Plan

Each of these daily plans is arranged according to the season. You can begin anywhere, but many of the items are calculated (when possible) according to temperatures and seasons in the United States.

Week 1: Summer Menu Option

Day 1:

Breakfast: Broccoli Cheese Omelet: 4 servings (+) 229 calories
Lunch: Arugula Salad: 4 servings (+) 257 calories
Dinner: Feta Chicken Burgers: 6 servings (+) 356 calories
Snack or Dessert: Strawberry Rhubarb Smoothie: 1 serving (+) 295 calories

Day 2:

Breakfast: Egg White Scramble with Cherry Tomatoes & Spinach:
4 servings (+) 142 calories
Lunch: Cucumber Salad: 4 servings (+) 68 calories
Dinner: Baked Salmon with Dill: 4 servings (+) 251 calories
Snack or Dessert: Fruit - Veggie & Cheese Board: 4 servings (+) 213 calories

Day 3:

Breakfast: Peanut Butter & Banana Greek Yogurt Bowl: 4 servings (+) 370 calories
Lunch: Feta Frittata: 2 servings (+) 203 calories
Dinner: Italian Chicken Skillet: 4 servings (+) 515 calories
Snack or Dessert: Honey Lime Fruit Salad: 8 servings (+) 115 calories

Day 4:

Breakfast: Poached Eggs: 2 servings (+) 72 calories
Lunch: Grecian Pasta Chicken Skillet: 4 servings (+) 373 calories
Dinner: Rosemary Thyme Lamb Chops: 4 servings (+) 231 calories
Snack or Dessert: Garlic Garbanzo Bean Spread: 2 tbsp. servings (+) 114 calories (Add your favorite crackers.)

Day 5:

Breakfast: Prosciutto - Lettuce - Tomato & Avocado Sandwiches: 4 servings (+) 240 calories
Lunch: Insalata Caprese II Salad: 6 servings (+) 311 calories
Dinner: Tomato Feta Salad: 4 servings (+) 121 calories
Snack or Dessert: Watermelon Cubes: 16 servings (+) 7 calories

Day 6:

Breakfast: Scrambled Eggs with Spinach – Tomato & Feta: 1-2
servings (+) 216 calories
Lunch: Quinoa Fruit Salad: 4 servings (+) 206 calories
Dinner: Lemon Chicken Skewers: 6 servings (+) 219 calories
Snack or Dessert: Chilled Dark Chocolate Fruit Kebabs: 6 servings (+) 254 calories

Day 7:

Breakfast: Spinach Omelet: 4 servings (+) 295 calories
Lunch: Shrimp Orzo Salad: 8 servings (+) 397 calories
Dinner: Summertime Mixed Spice Burgers: 6 servings (+) 192 calories

Snack or Dessert: Mango Pear Smoothie: 1 serving (+) 293 calories

Week 2

Day 8:

Breakfast: Avocado & Egg Breakfast Sandwich: 2 servings (+) 309 calories
Lunch: Avocado & Tuna Tapas: 4 servings (+) 294 calories
Dinner: Slow Cooked Lemon Chicken: 6 servings (+) 336 calories
Snack or Dessert: Honey Nut Granola: 6 servings (+) 337 calories

Day 9:

Breakfast: Baked Ricotta & Pears: 4 servings (+) 312 calories
Lunch: Roasted Tomato Pita Pizzas: 6 servings (+) 259 calories
Dinner: Herb-Crusted Halibut: 4 servings (+) 273 calories
Snack or Dessert: Kale Chips: 4 servings (+) 56 calories

Day 10:

Breakfast: Feta & Quinoa Egg Muffins: 12 servings (+) 113 calories
Lunch: Greek Lentil Soup: 4 servings (+) 357 calories
Dinner: Braised Chicken & Artichoke Hearts: 4 servings (+) 707 calories
Snack or Dessert: Walnut & Date Smoothie: 2 servings (+) 385 calories

Day 11:

Breakfast: Mashed Chickpea - Feta & Avocado Toast: 4 servings (+) 337 calories
Lunch: Cannellini Bean Lettuce Wraps: 4 servings (+) 211 calories
Dinner: Marinated Tuna Steak: 4 servings (+) 200 calories
Snack or Dessert: Italian Vanilla Greek Yogurt

Affogato: 4 servings (+) 270 calories

Day 12:

Breakfast: Ham & Egg Cups: 8 servings (+) 145 calories
Lunch: Stuffed Bell Peppers: 6 servings (+) 210 calories
Dinner: Penne with Shrimp: 8 servings (+) 385 calories
Snack or Dessert: Strawberry Greek Frozen Yogurt: 1 quart (+) 86 calories

Day 13:

Breakfast: Pumpkin Pancakes: 6 servings (+) 278 calories
Lunch: Mushroom Risotto: 4 servings (+) 322 calories
Dinner: Pan Seared Salmon: 4 servings (+) 371 calories
Snack or Dessert: Spiced Sweet Roasted Red Pepper Hummus: 8 servings (+) 64 calories (Add your favorite veggies.)

Day 14:

Breakfast: Scrambled Eggs With Goat Cheese & Roasted Pepper: 4 servings (+) 201 calories
Lunch: Stuffed Sweet Potatoes: 4 servings (+) 142.5 calories
Dinner: Speedy Tilapia With Avocado & Red Onion: 4 servings (+) 200 calories
Snack or Dessert: Honey Rosemary Almonds: 6 servings (+) 149 calories

Week 3

Day 15:

Breakfast: Christmas Breakfast Sausage Casserole: 8 servings (+) 377 calories
Lunch: Chicken Marrakesh: 8 servings (+) 290 calories
Dinner: Nicoise-Style Tuna Salad With Olives & White Beans: 4 servings (+) 548 calories
Snack or Dessert: Chocolate Avocado Pudding: 4 servings (+) 295.3 calories

Day 16:

Breakfast: Barley Porridge: 4 servings (+) 354 calories
Lunch: Cucumber Dill Greek Yogurt Salad: 6 servings (+) 49.6 calories
Dinner: Mediterranean Pork Chops: 4 servings (+) 161 calories
Snack or Dessert: Banana Sour Cream Bread: 32 servings (+) 263 calories

Day 17:

Breakfast: French Toast Delight: 12 servings (+) 123 calories
Lunch: Chicken & White Bean Soup: 6 servings (+) 248 calories
Dinner: Beef Cacciatore: 6 servings (+) 510 calories
Snack or Dessert: Chia Greek Yogurt Pudding: 4 servings (+) 263 calories

Day 18:

Breakfast: Crustless Spinach Quiche: 6 servings (+) 309 calories
Lunch: Italian Tuna Sandwiches: 4 servings (+) 347 calories
Dinner: Sweet Sausage Marsala: 6 servings (+) 509

calories
Snack or Dessert: Italian Apple Olive Oil Cake: 12 servings (+) 294 calories

Day 19:

Breakfast: Fruit Bulgur Breakfast Bowl: 6 servings (+) 301 calories
Lunch: Dill Salmon Salad Wraps: 6 servings (+) 336 calories
Dinner: Beef With Artichokes - Slow Cooker: 6 servings (+) 416 calories
Snack or Dessert: Maple Vanilla Baked Pears: 4 servings (+) 103.9 calories

Day 20:

Breakfast: Marinara Eggs With Parsley: 6 servings (+) 122 calories
Lunch: Fried Rice With Spinach - Peppers & Artichokes: 4 servings (+) 244 calories
Dinner: Slow Cooked Roasted Turkey Breast: 8 servings (+) 333 calories
Snack or Dessert: Olive Oil Chocolate Chip Cookies: 24 servings (+) 187 calories

Day 21:

Breakfast: Greek Yogurt Bowl With Peanut Butter & Bananas: 4 servings (+) 370 calories
Lunch: Mediterranean Bean Salad: 4 servings (+) 329 calories
Dinner: Spanish Moroccan Fish: 12 servings (+) 268 calories
Snack or Dessert: Mediterranean Flatbread: 6 servings (+) 450 calories

Week 4:

Day 22:

Breakfast: Greek Yogurt Breakfast Parfait with Roasted Grapes: 4 servings (+) 300 calories
Lunch: Chicken & Veggie Wraps: 4 servings (+) 278 calories
Dinner: Salmon With Warm Tomato-Olive Salad: 4 servings (+) 433 calories
Snack or Dessert: Roasted Peaches & Blueberries: 4 servings (+) 45.7 calories

Day 23:

Breakfast: Mediterranean Egg - Pepper & Mushroom Cup: 12 servings (+) 67 calories
Lunch: Greek Shrimp Farro Bowl: 2 servings (+) 428 calories
Dinner: Mussels With Olives & Potatoes: 4 servings (+) 345 calories
Snack or Dessert: Date Wraps: 16 servings (+) 35 calories

Day 24:

Breakfast: Artichoke Frittata: 4 servings (+) 199 calories
Lunch: Goat Cheese Salad: 4 servings (+) 322 calories
Dinner: Grilled Salmon: 4 servings (+) 214 calories
Snack or Dessert: Pistachio No-Bake Snack Bars: 8 servings (+) 220 calories

Day 25:

Breakfast: Greek Yogurt Pancakes: 6 servings (+) 258 calories
Lunch: Escarole with Garlic: 4 servings (+) 66 calories
Dinner: Chicken Thighs With Artichokes & Sun-Dried Tomatoes: 6 servings (+) 169 calories
Snack or Dessert: Mango Mousse: 4 servings (+) 358 calories

Day 26:

Breakfast: Overnight Blueberry French Toast: 10

servings (+) 485 calories

Lunch: Chickpea Salad: 4 servings (+) 163 calories

Dinner: Greek Honey & Lemon Pork Chops: 4 servings (+) 257 calories

Snack or Dessert: Yogurt & Olive Oil Brownies: 12 servings (+) 150 calories

Day 27:

Breakfast: Greek Egg Frittata: 6 servings (+) 107 calories
Lunch: Mediterranean Tuna Salad: 4 servings (+) 328 calories
Dinner: Greek Salad Tacos: 4 servings (+) 466 calories
Snack or Dessert: Sautéed Apricots: 4 servings (+) 207 calories

Day 28:

Breakfast: Roasted Asparagus Prosciutto & Egg: 4 servings (+) 199 calories
Lunch: Pasta With Sausage & Escarole: 4 servings (+) 333 calories
Dinner: Grilled Lamb Chops With Mint: 6 servings (+) 238 calories
Snack or Dessert: Almond-Stuffed Dates: 1 serving (+) 149 calories

Consider Adding Meal Prep for the Mediterranean Plan

Now that you have a great meal plan, you may decide it's time to consider doing a little bit of meal prep. This is especially true if you are just cooking for one or two people. Most recipes have four servings or more in them. You can start small by using a few essential products. You can save a ton of money by storing the extra food in the freezer to use at a later time when you just don't have time to prepare a meal from scratch.

Do you want to prepare all of the chicken, pork or other meal selections one night and the veggies the next night? Or: Do you want to cook each meal individually but in bulk? Either way, these are a few of the items to help you begin:

- Ziploc-type freezer bags
- Mason Jars – Pint or quart sized
- Rubbermaid Stackable - Glad Containers

The main thing to remember is to purchase items that are stackable, reusable, BPA-free, freezer safe, and microwavable. Choose a time when you won't be interrupted. Try to find meat and dairy that has an expiration date for as far in the future as possible. These choices will tend to remain fresh and last longer. This also applies to the "sell by" dates. The further in the future, either of these dates is, the surer you can be that the food is going to last the week. Dice or chop your own meats and vegetables and stop paying for the convenience.

Look Ahead For Emergencies:

- Prepare and freeze plenty of healthy fruits and yogurt into a delicious smoothie for the entire week. Enjoy one for breakfast or any time you have the craving. Chop your veggies in advance.

- As you prep, include lean proteins for the weekends in a container for a quick grab and go snack or luncheon for a weekend journey.

- Purchase foods in bulk to be used for taco meats, breakfast burritos, fajita fillings, soups, egg muffins, and so much more.

You will help eliminate stress. You will also love the fact that these foods will be ready when you are!

Chapter 6: Recipes for the Summer

Breakfast for Summer

Broccoli & Cheese Omelet

Serving Yields: 4
Nutritional Calorie Count: 229

Ingredients Needed:
- Fresh broccoli florets - 2.5 cups
- Large eggs - 6
- 2% milk - .25 cup
- Salt - .5 tsp.
- Pepper - .25 tsp.
- Grated Romano cheese - .33 cup
- Sliced pitted Greek olives - 33 cup
- Olive oil - 1 tbsp.
- To Garnish: Shaved Romano cheese & Minced fresh parsley
- Also Needed: 10-inch ovenproof skillet

Preparation Instructions:
1. Set the oven temperature to broil.
2. Place a steamer basket in a saucepan in about 1 inch of water. Toss the broccoli into the basket. Wait for it to boil.
3. Lower the heat to simmer for four to six minutes with a lid on.
4. Whisk the eggs, milk, salt, and pepper. Fold in the broccoli, olives, and grated cheese.
5. Prepare the skillet using the medium heat setting and add the oil. Fold in the egg mixture and cook for 6 minutes.
6. Place the skillet in the oven approximately 3-4 inches from the heat. Bake for 2-4 minutes or until the eggs are

set.
7. Transfer to the countertop to cool for about 5 minutes.
8. Slice into wedges. Sprinkle with the parsley and shaved cheese.

Egg White Scramble with Cherry Tomatoes & Spinach

Serving Yields: 4
Nutritional Calorie Count: 142

Ingredients Needed:

- Olive oil - 1 tbsp.
- Eggs - 1 whole & 10 egg whites
- Black pepper - .25 tsp.
- Salt - .5 tsp.
- Minced garlic clove - 1
- Halved cherry tomatoes - 2 cups
- Packed fresh baby spinach - 2 cups
- Light cream or Half & Half - .5 cup
- Finely grated parmesan cheese - .25 cup

Preparation Instructions:

1. Whisk the eggs, pepper, salt, and milk.
2. Prepare a skillet using the med-hi heat setting.
3. Toss in the garlic when the pan is hot. Sauté for approximately 30 seconds.
4. Pour in the tomatoes and spinach. Continue sautéing for one additional minute. The tomatoes should be softened and the spinach wilted.
5. Add the egg mixture into the pan using the medium heat setting. Fold the egg gently as it cooks for about two to three minutes.
6. Remove from the burner, and sprinkle with a sprinkle of cheese.

Peanut Butter & Banana Greek Yogurt Bowl

Serving Yields: 4
Nutritional Calorie Count: 370

Ingredients Needed:

- Medium bananas - 2
- Flaxseed meal - .25 cup
- Nutmeg - 1 tsp.
- Peanut butter - .25 cup
- Greek yogurt - vanilla - 4 cups

Preparation Instructions:

1. Peel and slice the bananas. Divide the yogurt amongst four serving dishes. Top each one off with sliced bananas.
2. Microwave the peanut butter for 30 to 40 seconds until completely melted.
3. Drizzle the peanut butter over the banana slices and sprinkle with the flaxseed meal. Top it off with the nutmeg and serve.

Poached Eggs

Serving Yields: 2
Nutritional Calorie Count: 72

Ingredients Needed:

- Salt - .5 tsp.
- Champagne vinegar - 1 tsp.
- Fresh eggs - 2

Preparation Instructions:

1. Prepare a saucepan with cold water and bring it to a boil using the medium temperature setting. Stir in the salt and vinegar.
2. Break each of the eggs into a ramekin. Place it close to the water and slide it out of the dish. Simmer until set.
3. Use a slotted spoon to lift it from the pan to help prevent sticking. Continue cooking until the yolk is runny and the white is cooked or about six minutes.
4. Prepare a container with ice water. Transfer the eggs from the pan to the bowl of ice water (It slows and stops the cooking process.)
5. Remove from the pan and drain on a paper towel before serving.

Prosciutto – Lettuce – Tomato & Avocado Sandwiches

Serving Yields: 4
Nutritional Calorie Count: 240

Ingredients Needed:

- Whole grain or whole wheat bread slices - 8
- Freshly ground black pepper - .25 tsp.
- Ripe avocado - 1 cut in half
- Kosher or sea salt - .25 tsp.
- Romaine lettuce - 4 full leaves
- Large ripe tomato - 1
- Prosciutto - 2 oz. - 8 thin slices

Preparation Instructions:

1. Tear the lettuce leaves into 8 pieces (total). Slice the tomato into two 8 rounds. Toast the bread and place it on a plate.
2. Use a spoon to remove the avocado flesh from the skin. Add it to a bowl. Sprinkle with the salt and pepper.
3. Whisk or gently mash the avocado until it's creamy. Spread over the bread.
4. Make one sandwich. Take a slice of avocado toast; top it with a lettuce leaf, a prosciutto slice, and a tomato slice. Top with another slice of lettuce tomato and continue. Repeat until all ingredients are made for four sandwiches.

Scrambled Eggs with Spinach – Tomato & Feta

Serving Yields: 1-2
Nutritional Calorie Count: 216

Ingredients Needed:

- Tomato – .5 of 1 - .33 cup
- Vegetable oil - 1 tbsp.
- Baby spinach - 1 cup
- Eggs - 3
- Pepper and salt - as desired
- Feta cheese - 2 tbsp.

Preparation Instructions:

1. Remove the seeds and dice the tomatoes. Cut the feta into cubes.
2. Warm up a skillet using the medium heat setting.
3. Sauté the spinach and tomatoes.
4. Once the spinach has wilted, whisk and stir in the eggs.
5. Scramble until done and give it a dusting of the salt and pepper.

Spinach Omelet

Serving Yields: 4
Nutritional Calorie Count: 295

Ingredients Needed:

- Olive oil - 3 tbsp.
- Small onion - 1
- Garlic clove - 1
- Large tomatoes - 4
- Eggs - 8
- Black pepper - .25 tsp.
- Fine sea salt - 1 tsp.
- Feta cheese - 2 oz.
- Flat leaf parsley - 1 tbsp.

Preparation Instructions:

1. Core and chop the tomatoes, parsley, and onion.
2. Warm up the oven to reach 400° Fahrenheit.
3. Pour the oil into an ovenproof skillet using high heat. Toss in the onions. Sauté until softened (5-7 min.).
4. Pour in the tomatoes, garlic, salt, and pepper.
5. Sauté for five more minutes and add the whisked eggs. Stir and cook for 3 to 5 minutes. When the bottom is set, put the skillet into the hot oven. Continue cooking for 5 additional minutes.
6. Transfer to the countertop and top it off with the parsley and feta. Serve warm.

Lunch Options for the Summer

Arugula Salad

Serving Yields: 4
Nutritional Calorie Count: 257

Ingredients Needed:

- Arugula leaves - 4 cups
- Cherry tomatoes - 1 cup
- Pine nuts - .25 cup
- Rice vinegar - 1 tbsp.
- Grape seed or olive oil - 2 tbsp.
- Pepper & Salt - to your liking
- Grated parmesan cheese - .25 cup
- Large avocado - 1 sliced

Preparation Instructions:

1. Rinse and dry the arugula leaves, grate the cheese, and slice the cherry tomatoes into halves. Peel and slice the avocado.
2. Combine the arugula, pine nuts, tomatoes, oil, vinegar, and cheese.
3. Sprinkle with a dusting of pepper and salt as desired.
4. Cover and toss to mix. Portion onto plates with the avocado slices, and enjoy.

Cucumber Salad

Serving Yields: 4
Nutritional Calorie Count: 68

Ingredients Needed:

- Cucumbers - 5-6
- Plain Greek yogurt - 8 oz.
- Garlic cloves - 2
- Oregano - 1 tsp.
- Fresh mint - 1 tbsp.
- Black pepper and Fine sea salt - .125 tsp. each

Preparation Instructions:

1. Use a sharp paring knife to slice the cucumbers. Mince the mint and garlic.
2. Mix the oregano, mint, garlic, yogurt, with the cucumbers in a mixing bowl. Sprinkle the cucumbers with the pepper and salt.
3. Place in the refrigerator for approximately one hour before your meal.

Feta Frittata

Serving Yields: 2
Nutritional Calorie Count: 203

Ingredients Needed:

- Green onion - 1
- Small garlic clove - 1
- Large eggs - 2
- Egg substitute - .5 cup
- Crumbled feta cheese - divided - 4 tbsp.
- Plum tomato - .33 cup
- Avocado slices - 4 thin
- Reduced-fat sour cream - 2 tbsp.
- Also Needed: 6-inch nonstick skillet

Preparation Instructions:

1. Thinly slice the onion and mince the garlic clove, chop the tomato, and peel the avocado before slicing.
2. Warm up the pan using the medium temperature setting and lightly spritz it with cooking oil.
3. Whisk the egg substitute, eggs, and three tablespoons of the feta cheese.
4. Add the egg mixture into the pan. Cover and simmer for 4 to 6 minutes.
5. Sprinkle with the rest of the feta cheese and tomato. Cover and continue cooking until the eggs are set or about 2 to 3 more minutes.
6. Let it rest for about 5 minutes before cutting it into halves. Serve with the avocado and sour cream.

Grecian Pasta Chicken Skillet

Serving Yields: 4 - 1.5 cups each
Nutritional Calorie Count: 373

Ingredients Needed:

- Reduced-sodium chicken broth - 1 can - 14.5 oz.
- Diced tomatoes undrained - no salt added - 1 can - 14.5 oz.
- Chicken breast - cut into 1-inch pieces - .75 lb.
- Water or white wine - .5 cup
- Garlic - 1 clove
- Dried oregano - .5 tsp.
- Multigrain thin spaghetti - 4 oz.
- Marinated and quartered artichoke hearts - 7.5 oz. jar
- Roasted sweet bell pepper strips - .25 cup
- Sliced ripe olives - .25 cup
- Baby spinach - 2 cups
- Chopped green onion - 1
- Fresh parsley - 2 tbsp.
- Lemon juice - 2 tbsp.
- Grated lemon zest - .5 tsp.
- Olive oil - 1 tbsp.
- Pepper - .5 tsp.
- Optional: Crumbled reduced-fat feta cheese to your liking

Preparation Instructions:

1. Drain and coarsely chop the artichoke hearts.
2. Combine the water/wine, chicken, garlic, oregano, chicken broth, and tomatoes in a large skillet.
3. Toss in the spaghetti and boil for 5-7 minutes. Simmer until the pink is removed from the chicken.
4. Stir in the spinach, pepper, oil, parsley, green onion, olives, red peppers, and the juice and zest of lemon.

5. Simmer for another 2-3 minutes or until the spinach is wilted.
6. Sprinkle with the cheese and serve.

Insalata Caprese II Salad

Serving Yields: 6
Nutritional Calorie Count: 311

Ingredients Needed:

- Large ripened tomato - .25-inches thick - 4
- Mozzarella cheese - .25-inches thick - 1 lb.
- Fresh basil leaves - .33 cup
- Extra-virgin olive oil - 3 tbsp.
- Fine sea salt - as desired
- Freshly cracked black pepper - as desired

Preparation Instructions:

1. Prepare the salad by alternating and overlapping tomato slices with mozzarella cheese and the basil leaves.
2. Spritz with the olive oil and dust with a portion of the pepper and salt. Serve.

Quinoa Fruit Salad

Serving Yields: 4
Nutritional Calorie Count: 206

Ingredients Needed:

- Raw honey - 2 tbsp.
- Fresh strawberries - 1 cup
- Fresh lime juice - 2 tbsp.
- Cooked quinoa - 1 cup
- Diced mango - 1
- Fresh blackberries - 1 cup
- Diced peach - 1
- Fresh basil - 1 tsp.
- Kiwi - 2

Preparation Instructions:

1. Slice the strawberries and dice the peach and mango.
2. Combine the basil, honey, and lime juice.
3. In another bowl, mix the mango, kiwi, peach, blackberries, quinoa, and the strawberries.
4. Stir in the honey mixture and toss well before serving.

Shrimp Orzo Salad

Serving Yields: 8
Nutritional Calorie Count: 397 - per 1.5 cup serving

Ingredients Needed:

- Orzo pasta - 16 oz. 1 pkg.
- Cooked shrimp - .75 lb.
- Water-packed artichoke hearts - 14 oz. can
- Sweet red pepper - 1 cup
- Red onion - .75 cup
- Green pepper - 1 cup
- Pitted Greek olives - .5 cup
- Freshly minced parsley - .5 cup
- Freshly chopped dill - .33 cup
- Greek vinaigrette - .75 cup

Preparation Instructions:

1. Peel and devein the shrimp and cook. Slice each one into thirds (31-40-count). Finely chop the onions and peppers.
2. Prepare the orzo according to the package instructions. Drain and rinse the orzo with cold water. Drain well.
3. Combine the shrimp, orzo, olives, herbs, and veggies.
4. Sprinkle with vinaigrette and toss to coat.
5. Refrigerate and cover until ready to serve.
6. Serve as a delicious side salad.

Dinner Specialties for the Summer

Baked Salmon with Dill

Serving Yields: 4
Nutritional Calorie Count: 251

Ingredients Needed:

- Salmon fillets - 4- 6 oz. portions - 1-inch thick
- Finely chopped fresh dill - 1.5 tbsp.
- Black pepper -.125 tsp.
- Kosher salt - .5 tsp.
- Lemon wedges - 4

Preparation Instructions:

1. Warm up the oven to reach 350° Fahrenheit.
2. Grease a baking tin with a spritz of cooking oil spray and add the fish.
3. Lightly spritz the fish with the spray along with a shake of the salt, pepper, and dill.
4. Bake for ten minutes or until the fish is easily flaked with a fork.
5. Serve with the lemon wedges.

Feta Chicken Burgers

Serving Yields: 6
Nutritional Calorie Count: 356 with 1 tbsp. sauce

Ingredients Needed:

- Reduced-fat mayonnaise - .25 cup
- Finely chopped cucumber - .25 cup
- Black pepper - .25 tsp.
- Garlic powder - 1 tsp.
- Chopped roasted sweet red pepper - .5 cup
- Greek seasoning - .5 tsp.
- Lean ground chicken - 1.5 lb.
- Crumbled feta cheese - 1 cup
- Whole wheat burger buns - 6 toasted

Preparation Instructions:

1. Warm up the broiler to the oven ahead of time. Combine the mayonnaise and cucumber together. Set aside.
2. Combine all of the seasonings and the red pepper for the burgers. Work in the chicken and the cheese. Shape into 6 - ½-inch thick patties.
3. Broil the burgers approximately four inches from the heat source. It should take about 3-4 minutes on each side until the thermometer reaches 165° Fahrenheit.
4. Serve on the buns with the cucumber sauce. Top it off with tomato and lettuce if desired and serve.

Italian Chicken Skillet

Serving Yields: 4
Nutritional Calorie Count: 515

Ingredients Needed:

- Olive oil - 1 tbsp.
- Chicken breast halves - 4
- Garlic - 2 cloves
- Red cooking wine - .5 cup
- Italian style diced tomatoes - 28 oz. can
- Seashell pasta - 8 oz.
- Freshly chopped spinach - 5 oz.
- Shredded mozzarella cheese - 1 cup

Preparation Instructions:

1. Warm up a large skillet and add the oil.
2. Add the chicken and simmer for about five to eight minutes.
3. Pour in the diced tomatoes and wine. Let it come to a boil using the high heat setting.
4. Stir in the pasta. Leave the top off and continue cooking. Stir occasionally until the shells are thoroughly cooked (10 min. after the pasta starts boiling).
5. Spread the spinach over top of the pasta and cover. The spinach should be ready in about 5 minutes.
6. Sprinkle with the cheese and simmer for another five minutes or until the cheese is bubbling.

Lemon Chicken Skewers

Serving Yields: 6
Nutritional Calorie Count: 219

Ingredients Needed:

- Olive oil - .25 cup
- Lemon juice - 3 tbsp.
- White wine vinegar - 1 tbsp.
- Grated lemon zest - 2 tsp.
- Salt - 1 tsp.
- Dried oregano - .25 tsp.
- Freshly cracked black pepper - .25 tsp.
- Sugar - .5 tsp.
- Zucchini - 3 medium - 1.5-inch slices
- Minced garlic - 2 cloves
- Medium onions - 3 into wedges
- Cherry tomatoes - 12
- Chicken breasts - 1.5 lb.

Preparation Instructions:

1. Cut the zucchini in half lengthwise and slice into 1.5-inch slices.
2. Peel the onions and cut into wedges. Zest the lemon. Cut the chicken into 1.5-inch pieces.
3. Prepare the marinade; combine the sugar, pepper, oregano, salt, lemon zest, vinegar, lemon juice, and oil - reserving .25 cup for basting.
4. Fold in the chicken and toss to cover.
5. Add the rest of the marinade in a mixing container and add the tomatoes, onions, and zucchini. Cover and place in the fridge overnight (for best results) or a minimum of four hours.
6. When ready to cook, drain and trash the marinade.
7. Soak the wooden skewers in water.

8. Thread the chicken and veggies onto the soaked skewers.
9. Place the skewers on the grill for six minutes using the medium heat setting. It's done when poked with a fork - the juices will run clear.

Rosemary Thyme Lamb Chops

Serving Yields: 4
Nutritional Calorie Count: 231

Ingredients Needed:

- Lamb loin chops - 8 - 3 oz. each
- Salt - .25 tsp.
- Pepper - .5 tsp.
- Dijon mustard - 3 tbsp.
- Fresh rosemary - 1 tbsp.
- Garlic - 3 cloves
- Fresh thyme - 1 tbsp.

Preparation Instructions:

1. Mince the thyme and garlic.
2. Combine the mustard, garlic, rosemary, and thyme in a mixing container. Sprinkle the lamb chops with the pepper and salt.
3. Lightly grease the grill rack. Prepare the chops on the grill using the medium heat setting for 6-8 minutes. For Doneness: Med-well is 145° Fahrenheit, the medium is 140° Fahrenheit, and well-done is at 135° Fahrenheit.

Summertime Mixed Spice Burgers

Serving Yields: 6
Nutritional Calorie Count: 192

Ingredients Needed:

- Finely chopped medium onion - 1
- Freshly minced parsley - 3 tbsp.
- Clove of garlic - 1 minced
- Ground allspice - .75 tsp.
- Pepper - .75 tsp.
- Ground nutmeg - .25 tsp.
- Cinnamon - .5 tsp.
- Salt - .5 tsp.
- Fresh mint - 2 tbsp.
- 90% lean ground beef - 1.5 lb.
- Tzatziki sauce - optional

Preparation Instructions:

1. Whisk the nutmeg, salt, cinnamon, pepper, allspice, garlic cloves, minced mint, parsley, and the onion.
2. Add the beef and prepare (6) 2 by 4-inch oblong patties.
3. Use the medium heat setting to grill the patties or broil four inches from the heat source for four to six minutes per side.
4. When it's done, the meat thermometer will register 160° Fahrenheit. Serve with the sauce if desired.

Tomato Feta Salad

Serving Yields: 4
Nutritional Calorie Count: 121

Ingredients Needed:

- Balsamic vinegar - 2 tbsp.
- Freshly minced basil - 1.5 tsp. or .5 tsp. dried
- Salt -.5 tsp.
- Coarsely chopped sweet onion - .5 cup
- Olive oil - 2 tbsp.
- Cherry or grape tomatoes - 1 lb.
- Crumbled feta cheese - .25 cup.

Preparation Instructions:

1. Whisk the salt, basil, and vinegar.
2. Toss the onion into the vinegar mixture, and let it rest for about 5 minutes
3. Slice the tomatoes into halves and stir in the tomatoes, feta cheese, and oil type evenly. Serve.

Snacks for the Summer

Chilled Dark Chocolate Fruit Kebabs

Serving Yields: 6
Nutritional Calorie Count: 254

Ingredients Needed:

- Hulled strawberries - 12
- Green or red seedless grapes - 24
- Pitted cherries - 12
- Blueberries - 24
- Dark chocolate - 8 oz.

Preparation Instructions:

1. Prepare a rimmed baking sheet with a layer of parchment paper. Lay out six 12-inch skewers. Prepare the skewers with the fruit - alternating each flavor.
2. Use a microwave-safe dish to heat the chocolate on high for one minute. Stir to melt the chocolate.
3. Add the melted chocolate to a plastic sandwich bag and twist a corner. Snip the corner off of the bag to use as a pipe. Squeeze the bag to drizzle the chocolate over the kebabs.
4. Arrange the sheet in the freezer to chill for 20 minutes before serving.

Fruit – Veggie & Cheese Board

Serving Yields: 4
Nutritional Calorie Count: 213

Ingredients Needed:

- Sliced fruits - Peaches, plums, pears, or apples - 2 cups
- Finger food fruits - Figs, grapes, cherries, or berries - 2 cups
- Raw veggies cut into sticks - Cauliflower, broccoli, celery, or carrots
- Jarred, canned, or cured veggies - Artichoke hearts, roasted Peppers or 0.5 cup of olives
- Cubed cheese - Gorgonzola, goat cheese, Asiago, or feta - Approximately 6 oz. or 1 cup

Preparation Instructions:

1. Prep the produce: Wash all of the veggies and slice into bite-size pieces.
2. Arrange all of the fixings on a wooden board or a serving tray. You can also cover a baking tin with parchment paper.
3. Add small spoons and little forks for the berries and olives and a knife for cutting the cheese.
4. Serve with small individual plates and napkins.

Garlic Garbanzo Bean Spread

Serving Yields: 1.5 cups
Nutritional Calorie Count: 114 per 2 tbsp. serving

Ingredients Needed:

- Chickpeas or garbanzo beans - 1 can - 15 oz.
- Olive oil - .5 cup
- Green onion - 1 - into 3 pieces
- Lemon juice - 1 tbsp.
- Garlic cloves - 1-2 peeled
- Salt - .25 tsp.
- Freshly minced parsley - 2 tbsp.
- Baked pita chips and assorted fresh veggies
- Also Needed: Food Processor

Preparation Instructions:

1. Combine the chickpeas or garbanzo beans, oil, parsley, lemon juice, garlic, salt, and green onion.
2. Add the ingredients into the blender and process until mixed.
3. Empty into a dish and refrigerate until ready to serve.
4. Enjoy with the pita chips and veggies.

Honey Lime Fruit Salad

Serving Yields: 8
Nutritional Calorie Count: 115

Ingredients Needed:

- Sliced bananas - 2 large
- Fresh blueberries - .5 lb.
- Fresh strawberries - 1 lb.
- Honey - 2 tbsp.
- Lime - 1 juiced
- Pine nuts - .33 cup

Preparation Instructions:

1. Hull and slice the strawberries and bananas.
2. Combine the blueberries, strawberries, and bananas in a bowl.
3. Cross over with the lime juice and honey.
4. Stir well and sprinkle with the nuts before serving.

Strawberry Greek Frozen Yogurt

Serving Yields: 1 quart
Nutritional Calorie Count: 86

Ingredients Needed:

- 2% plain Greek yogurt - 3 cups
- Fresh lemon juice - .25 cup
- Sugar - 1 cup
- Vanilla - 2 tsp.
- Salt - .125 tsp.
- Sliced strawberries - 1 cup
- Also Needed: 1.5 to 2-quart ice cream maker

Preparation Instructions:

1. Whisk the vanilla, salt, lemon juice, yogurt, and sugar until creamy.
2. Place the mixture in the ice cream maker. Prepare according to the manufacturer's directions.
3. Toss in the sliced berries for the last minute of the cycle.
4. Empty into a container and freeze for two to four hours before serving.
5. Let the ice cream sit out at room temperature for about 5 to 15 minutes before serving for best results.

Watermelon Cubes

Serving Yields: 16
Nutritional Calorie Count: 7

Ingredients Needed:

- Seedless watermelon cubes - 16 - 1-inch
- Finely chopped cucumber - .33 cup
- Finely chopped red onion - 5 tsp.
- Minced fresh mint - 2 tsp.
- Lime juice - .5 - 1 tsp. lime juice
- Freshly minced cilantro - 2 tsp.

Preparation Instructions:

1. Use a measuring spoon or a small melon baller to remove the center of each of the watermelon cubes. Leave a ¼-inch shell. Use the pulp another time.
2. In a small dish, mix the remaining fixings. Spoon into the watermelon cubes and serve.

Smoothies

Mango Pear Smoothie

Serving Yields: 1
Nutritional Calorie Count: 293

Ingredients Needed:

- Plain Greek yogurt - .5 cup
- Ice cubes - 2
- Mango - .5 of 1
- Kale - 1 cup
- Ripened pear - 1

Preparation Instructions:

1. Combine each of the ingredients in a blender.
2. Mix well until thickened and smooth.
3. Serve in a chilled glass.

Strawberry Rhubarb Smoothie

Serving Yields: 1
Nutritional Calorie Count: 295

Ingredients Needed:

- Sliced strawberries - 1 cup
- Chopped rhubarb - 1 stalk
- Raw honey - 2 tbsp.
- Ice cubes - 3
- Ground cinnamon - .125 tsp.
- Plain Greek yogurt - .5 cup

Preparation Instructions:

1. Pour water into a small saucepan and add the rhubarb. Boil for 3 minutes before draining and adding to a blender.
2. Prepare the rest of the fixings and add to the blender along with the honey, yogurt, cinnamon, and ice.
3. Blend well until creamy smooth, serving a chilled glass.

Chapter 7: Recipes for the Fall & Autumn Months

Breakfast Favorites for Fall/Autumn

Avocado & Egg Breakfast Sandwich

Serving Yields: 2
Nutritional Calorie Count: 309

Ingredients Needed:

- Toasted bread slices - whole wheat - 4
- Pitted avocado - 1
- Steamed asparagus spears - 8-12
- Sliced hard-boiled egg - 1
- Olive oil - as needed
- Freshly ground pepper & coarse sea salt - as desired
- Optional: Dijon mustard

Preparation Instructions:

1. Peel and mash the avocado. Toast the bread.
2. Prepare the sandwich by using the mustard with a layer of the avocado.
3. Add the asparagus spears and eggs.
4. Give it a drizzle of oil along with some salt and pepper. Close and serve.

Baked Ricotta & Pears

Serving Yields: 4
Nutritional Calorie Count: 312

Ingredients Needed:

- Ricotta cheese - whole-milk - 16 oz. container
- Large eggs - 2
- White whole wheat flour - .25 cup
- Sugar - 1 tbsp.
- Nutmeg - .25 tsp.
- Diced pear - 1
- Water - 2 tbsp.
- Vanilla extract - 1 tsp.
- Honey - 1 tbsp.
- Also Needed: 4 - 6 oz. ramekins

Preparation Instructions:

1. Heat up the oven to reach 400° Fahrenheit.
2. Lightly spray the ramekins with a spritz of cooking oil spray.
3. Whisk the flour, nutmeg, vanilla, sugar, eggs, and the ricotta together in a large mixing container.
4. Spoon the ingredients into the dishes. Bake for 20 to 25 minutes. The ricotta should be set. Take it out of the oven. Let it cool slightly.
5. In a saucepan, using the medium temperature setting, add the cored and diced pear into the water for about 10 minutes until slightly softened. Take the pan off of the burner and stir in the honey.
6. Serve the ricotta ramekins with the warm pear and enjoy.

Feta & Quinoa Egg Muffins

Serving Yields: 12
Nutritional Calorie Count: 113

Ingredients Needed:

- Cooked quinoa - 1 cup
- Chopped baby spinach - 2 cups
- Kalamata olives - .5 cup
- Tomatoes - 1 cup
- White onion - .5 cup
- Fresh oregano - 1 tbsp.
- Salt - .5 tsp.
- Olive oil - 2 tsp. (+) more for coating pans
- Eggs - 8
- Crumbled feta cheese - 1 cup
- Also Needed: 12-cup muffin tin

Preparation Instructions:

1. Warm up the oven to reach 350° Fahrenheit.
2. Lightly grease the muffin tray cups with a spritz of cooking oil.
3. Prepare a skillet using the medium heat setting and add the oil. When hot, toss in the onions and cook for two minutes.
4. Pour in the tomatoes and sauté one minute. Add the spinach and continue cooking for another minute or until the leaves have wilted.
5. Remove from the heat and add the oregano and olives. Set aside.
6. Crack the eggs into a bowl and blend using an immersion stick blender. Add the cooked veggies in with the remainder of the ingredients.
7. Stir until combined and spoon into the greased muffin cups.

8. Bake for 30 minutes until browned and the muffins are set.
9. Cool for 10 minutes.

Ham & Egg Cups

Serving Yields: 8
Nutritional Calorie Count: 145

Ingredients Needed:

- Cooked ham – deli style - 8 thin slices
- Mozzarella cheese - .25 cups or 1 oz.
- Eggs - 8
- Basil – optional - 8 tsp.
- Black pepper - as desired
- Grape or cherry tomatoes - 6 or as desired
- Also Needed: Muffin tin - 8-count

Preparation Instructions:

1. Program the oven setting to 350°F. Coat the muffin tin cups with the spray.
2. Press the ham slice into the bottom and add the cheese to each of the prepared cups. Break an egg into the cup and sprinkle with the pepper. Add the pesto, if using. Slice the tomatoes into halves, and place on each of the cups.
3. Bake 18-20 minutes. The egg whites should be set, similar to a regular poached egg. Leave them in the cups for 3-5 minutes. Then, carefully take the cups out of the tin and serve.

Mashed Chickpea – Feta & Avocado Toast

Serving Yields: 4
Nutritional Calorie Count: 337

Ingredients Needed:

- Chickpeas - 15 oz. can
- Diced feta cheese - 2 oz. - .5 cup
- Avocado - 1 pitted
- Fresh orange juice -1 tbsp. or lemon juice - 2 tsp.
- Freshly cracked black pepper - .5 tsp.
- Honey - 2 tsp.
- Multigrain toast - 4 slices

Preparation Instructions:

1. Toast the bread. Drain the chickpeas. Scoop the avocado flesh into the bowl.
2. Use a large fork or potato masher to mash them together until the mix is spreadable.
3. Pour in the lemon juice, pepper, and the feta.
4. Mix well and divide onto the four slices of toast. Drizzle with the honey and serve.

Pumpkin Pancakes

Serving Yields: 6
Nutritional Calorie Count: 278

Ingredients Needed:

- Milk - 1.5 cups
- Egg - 1
- Pumpkin puree - 1 cup
- Vegetable oil - 2 tbsp.
- Vinegar - 2 tbsp.
- Salt - .5 tsp.
- All-purpose flour - 2 cups
- Baking powder - 2 tsp.
- Ground allspice - 1 tsp.
- Brown sugar - 3 tbsp.
- Baking soda - 1 tsp.
- Cinnamon - 1 tsp.
- Ground ginger - .5 tsp.

Preparation Instructions:

1. Whisk the vinegar, oil, egg, pumpkin, and the milk together.
2. Combine the salt, ginger, cinnamon, allspice, baking soda, brown sugar, baking powder, and the flour in another bowl.
3. Stir the fixings together just enough to combine.
4. Warm up a frying pan or oiled griddle using the medium-high temperature setting.
5. Pour the batter into the griddle (for 6 servings) and brown on both sides. Serve hot.

Scrambled Eggs with Goat Cheese & Roasted Pepper

Serving Yields: 4
Nutritional Calorie Count: 201

Ingredients Needed:

- Extra-virgin olive oil - 1.5 tsp.
- Bell peppers - 1 medium pepper - 1 cup
- Garlic - 2 cloves - 1 tsp. minced
- Large eggs - 6
- Sea salt - .25 tsp.
- Water - 2 tbsp.
- Crumbled goat cheese - 2 oz. - .5 cup
- Loosely packed chopped fresh mint - 2 tbsp.

Preparation Instructions:

1. Use the medium-high heat setting to prepare a large skillet. Add the oil.
2. When hot, toss in the peppers and simmer for about five minutes. Stir in the garlic. Continue cooking for one minute.
3. Whisk the water, eggs, and salt in a mixing dish.
4. Reduce the temperature setting to med-low.
5. Pour in the egg mixture over top of the peppers. Simmer for one to two minutes until they're set on the bottom.
6. Sprinkle with the goat cheese and continue cooking for one to two more minutes. Stir until they are soft set. Garnish with the fresh mint and serve.

Lunch Options for Fall/Autumn

Avocado & Tuna Tapas

Serving Yields: 4
Nutritional Calorie Count: 294

Ingredients Needed:

- Solid white tuna packed in water - 12 oz. can
- Mayonnaise - 1 tbsp.
- Thinly sliced green onions - 3 (+) more for garnish
- Chopped red bell pepper - .5 of 1
- Garlic salt and black pepper - to taste
- Balsamic vinegar - 1 dash
- Ripe avocados - 2

Preparation Instructions:

1. Drain the tuna well. Chop the bell pepper, and thinly slice the onions. Remove the pit and slice the avocados into halves.
2. Whisk the vinegar, red pepper, onions, mayonnaise, and tuna.
3. Sprinkle with the salt and pepper.
4. Load the avocado halves with the tuna.
5. Top it off with a portion of green onions and black pepper. Serve.

Cannellini Bean Lettuce Wraps

Serving Yields: 4
Nutritional Calorie Count: 211 - 2 wraps per serving

Ingredients Needed:

- Extra-virgin olive oil - 1 tbsp.
- Red onion - .5 cup
- Tomatoes - 1 medium - .75 cup
- Freshly cracked black pepper - .25 tsp.
- Fresh curly parsley - .25 cup
- Great Northern beans or cannellini beans - 1 can - 15 oz.
- Prepared hummus - .5 cup
- Romaine lettuce leaves - 8

Preparation Instructions:

1. Drain and rinse the veggies and beans. Chop the tomatoes and onion into fine pieces.
2. Use the medium heat setting. Add the oil into a large skillet.
3. Toss in the onions and sauté for 3 minutes. Pour in the tomatoes and pepper. Simmer for three more minutes. Stir occasionally.
4. Pour in the drained beans and continue cooking for 3 additional minutes. Mix in the parsley after removing it from the burner.
5. Spread the hummus over each of the leaves of lettuce. Spread the bean mixture to the center of each leaf. Fold it over to make a wrap and serve.

Greek Lentil Soup

Serving Yields: 4
Nutritional Calorie Count: 357

Ingredients Needed:

- Brown lentils - 8 oz.
- Olive oil - .25 cup or as needed
- Minced garlic - 1 tbsp.
- Onion - 1
- Large carrot - 1
- Water - 1 quart
- Dried oregano - 1 pinch
- Crushed dried rosemary - 1 pinch
- Bay leaves - 2
- Tomato paste - 1 tbsp.
- Salt and ground black pepper - as desired
- Optional: Red wine vinegar - 1 tsp.

Preparation Instructions:

1. Mince the garlic and chop the onion and carrot.
2. Prep the lentils in a large saucepan with enough water to cover by about 1 inch. Once the beans start boiling, cook until tender or about ten minutes and drain in a colander.
3. Warm up the oil in a pan and using the medium heat setting. Toss in the onion, carrot, and garlic. Simmer approximately five minutes.
4. Pour in the water, lentils, oregano, bay leaves, and rosemary. Once boiling, reduce the temperature setting to med-low and cover. Cook for another ten minutes.
5. Sprinkle with the pepper and salt. Stir in the tomato paste.
6. Cover and simmer 30 to 40 minutes - stirring occasionally. Add water as needed.

7. When ready to serve, drizzle with the vinegar and one teaspoon of olive oil.

Mushroom Risotto

Serving Yields: 4
Nutritional Calorie Count: 322

Ingredients Needed:

- Olive oil - 2 tbsp.
- Thinly slice shallot - 1
- Large sliced mushrooms - 10
- Red wine - .5 cup
- Faro - 1 cup
- Vegetable broth - .5 cup or as needed
- Parmesan cheese - .5 cup
- Flat leaf parsley - 1 tbsp.
- Black pepper - .25 tsp.
- Fine sea salt - 1 tsp.

Preparation Instructions:

1. Place a skillet on a stovetop burner using the high heat setting.
2. Add the oil and shallot. Simmer for 3 to 5 minutes.
3. When the shallot is softened, pour in the red wine and mushrooms.
4. Add the faro. Simmer for approximately three minutes. Stir often until the broth is absorbed. Add more broth as needed. Continue until it's tender.
5. Take the skillet from the burner and add the parmesan, salt, pepper, and parsley.
6. Serve warm.

Roasted Tomato Pita Pizzas

Serving Yields: 6
Nutritional Calorie Count: 259

Ingredients Needed:

- Grape tomatoes - 2 pints or about 3 cups
- Garlic cloves - 2 minced
- Chopped fresh thyme leaves - 1 tsp. - 6 Sprigs
- Freshly cracked black pepper - .25 tsp.
- Shredded parmesan cheese - 3 oz. or .75 cup
- Kosher or sea salt - .25 tsp.
- Whole wheat pita bread - 6

Preparation Instructions:

1. Warm up the oven to reach 425° Fahrenheit.
2. Combined the tomatoes, salt, pepper, thyme, garlic, and oil. In a baking pan.
3. Roast for 10 minutes. Pull out the rack from the oven and stir the tomatoes with a wooden spoon or spatula. Mash down to soften the tomatoes and roast for another 10 minutes.
4. Prepare the pita bread with 2 tablespoons of cheese. Arrange them on a large rimmed baking sheet. Toast for the last 5 minutes of the cooking cycle.
5. Remove everything from the oven. Stir the tomatoes and spoon out about one-third of the sauce over each of the pita bread to serve.

Stuffed Bell Peppers

Serving Yields: 6
Nutritional Calorie Count: 210

Ingredients Needed:

- Uncooked bulgur - .5 cup
- Ground beef - 1 lb.
- Frozen chopped spinach - 10 oz. pkg.
- Medium red bell peppers - 3
- Grated zucchini - 2 cups
- Chopped tomatoes - 29 oz.
- Minced white onion - 1 cup
- Salt & black pepper - .5 tsp. each
- Dried oregano - .5 tsp.
- Egg - 1
- Crumbled feta cheese - .33 cup
- Also Needed: 9x13-inch baking dish

Preparation Instructions:

1. Thaw and squeeze the water out of the spinach. Core and slice the bell peppers into halves lengthwise. Chop the tomatoes. Grate the zucchini and mince the white onion.
2. Warm up the oven to reach 350° Fahrenheit.
3. Add all of the fixings except for the cheese, tomatoes, and pepper into a container and mix well.
4. Arrange the peppers in the baking dish (cut side up). Fill each of the halves with the prepared stuffing. Add the tomatoes and sprinkle with cheese.
5. Place a lid on the dish or cover with foil.
6. Bake for about half of an hour. Take the top off and bake until the top is browned (approx. 25 minutes).
7. Serve immediately.

Stuffed Sweet Potatoes

Serving Yields: 4
Nutritional Calorie Count: 142.5

Ingredients Needed:

- Small sweet potatoes - 4
- Cooked black beans - 15 oz.
- Corn - 1 cup
- Thinly sliced green onions - 3
- Chopped cilantro - .5 cup

Ingredients Needed For The Vinaigrette:

- Lime - 2 - juice and zest
- Salt and ground black pepper - .5 tsp. each
- Honey - 2 tsp.
- Adobo sauce - 2 tsp.
- Olive oil - 1 tbsp.

Preparation Instructions:

1. Set the oven temperature to 350° Fahrenheit.
2. Whisk each of the fixings in a mixing container until well-combined.
3. Arrange the sweet potatoes on a baking sheet. Bake for 45 to 60 minutes.
4. Stir together the cilantro, onion, corn, and the beans.
5. Pour in the prepared vinaigrette, and toss until combined.
6. Once the potatoes are done, slice into halves lengthwise and let them cool for approximately 15 minutes.
7. Push down the center of each one to create a divot. You can use the back of a spoon. Add the prepared corn mixture and serve.

Dinner Specialties for Fall/Autumn

Braised Chicken & Artichoke Hearts

Serving Yields: 4
Nutritional Calorie Count: 707

Ingredients Needed:

- Olive oil - 1 tbsp.
- Chicken legs - 4 quarters
- Yellow onion - 1
- Garlic - 4 cloves
- Black pepper - 1 tbsp.
- Red pepper flakes - .5 tsp.
- Salt - 1 tsp.
- Chicken stock or low-sodium broth - 1-quart
- Canned artichoke hearts - 10
- Cherry peppers - 2 cups
- Lemons - juiced - 2
- Fresh thyme sprigs - 8
- Butter beans - 16 oz. can
- Also Needed: Dutch oven

Preparation Instructions:

1. Dice the onion and garlic. Drain the butter beans. Drain the artichokes and cut them in half.
2. Warm up the oven to reach 375° Fahrenheit.
3. Prepare the pan using the high heat setting and add the oil.
4. Sear the chicken until browned or about 5 minutes on each side. Set aside on a warm platter.
5. Stir in the garlic, onion, pepper flakes, salt, and black pepper. Cook for about 1 minute. Stir in the broth and let

it simmer for another minute or so. Remove from the heat.
6. Put the chicken back in the Dutch oven and add the thyme, lemon juice, cherry peppers, and artichoke hearts.
7. Put the pan in the oven to bake for about one hour.
8. Take the chicken out of the cooker and place in a warm platter again.
9. Stir the beans into the pan with the broth and artichoke mixture.
10. Place each leg quarter in a serving dish. Add a ladle of the artichoke, bean, and broth mixture over each serving.

Herb-Crusted Halibut

Serving Yields: 4
Nutritional Calorie Count: 273

Ingredients Needed:

- Panko bread crumbs - .75 cup
- Fresh parsley - .33 cup
- Fresh dill - .25 cup
- Fresh chives - .25 cup
- Extra-virgin olive oil - 1 tbsp.
- Finely grated lemon zest - 1 tsp.
- Sea salt - 1 tsp.
- Ground black pepper - .25 tsp.
- Halibut fillets - 4 - 6 oz.

Preparation Instructions:

1. Chop the fresh dill, chives, and parsley. Line a baking sheet with a layer of foil.
2. Warm up the oven to reach 400° Fahrenheit.
3. Combine the salt, pepper, lemon zest, olive oil, chives, dill, parsley, and the breadcrumbs in a mixing bowl.
4. Rinse the halibut well. Use paper towels to dry before baking.
5. Arrange the fish on the baking sheet. Spoon the crumbs over the fish and press into each of the fillets.
6. Bake until the fish is easily flaked and the top is browned or about 10 to 15 minutes.

Marinated Tuna Steak

Serving Yields: 4
Nutritional Calorie Count: 200

Ingredients Needed:

- Olive oil - 2 tbsp.
- Orange juice - .25 cup
- Soy sauce - .25 cup
- Lemon juice - 1 tbsp.
- Fresh parsley - 2 tbsp.
- Garlic clove - 1
- Ground black pepper - .5 tsp.
- Fresh oregano - .5 tsp.
- Tuna steaks - 4 - 4 oz. steaks

Preparation Instructions:

1. Mince the garlic, and chop the oregano and parsley.
2. In a glass container, mix the pepper, oregano, garlic, parsley, lemon juice, soy sauce, olive oil, and orange juice.
3. Warm up the grill using the high heat setting. Grease the grate with oil.
4. Add to tuna steaks and cook for 5 to 6 minutes. Turn and baste with the marinated sauce.
5. Cook another 5 minutes or until it's the way you like it. Discard the remaining marinade.

Pan Seared Salmon

Serving Yields: 4
Nutritional Calorie Count: 371

Ingredients Needed:

- Salmon fillets - 4 - 6 oz. each
- Olive oil - 2 tbsp.
- Capers - 2 tbsp.
- Salt and Pepper - .125 tsp. each
- Lemon - 4 slices

Preparation Instructions:

1. Warm up a heavy skillet for about 3 minutes using the medium heat setting.
2. Lightly spritz the salmon with olive oil. Arrange in the pan and increase the temperature setting to high.
3. Sear for approximately three minutes. Sprinkle with the salt, pepper, and capers.
4. Flip the salmon over and continue cooking for 5 minutes or until browned the way you like it.
5. Garnish with lemon slices and serve.

Penne with Shrimp

Serving Yields: 8
Nutritional Calorie Count: 385

Ingredients Needed:

- Penne pasta - 16 oz. pkg.
- Salt - .25 tsp.
- Olive oil - 2 tbsp.
- Red onion - .25 cup
- Minced garlic - 1 tbsp.
- White wine - .25 cup
- Diced tomatoes - 2 - 14.5 oz. cans
- Shrimp - 1 lb.
- Grated parmesan cheese - 1 cup

Preparation Instructions:

1. Peel and devein the shrimp. Dice the red onion and garlic.
2. Add salt to a large pot of water. Place on the stovetop and set to boil. Add the pasta and cook for 9 to 10 minutes. Drain.
3. Empty the oil into a skillet. Warm up using the medium heat setting.
4. Stir in the garlic and onion. Sauté until tender and mix in the tomatoes and wine. Continue cooking about 10 minutes, stirring occasionally.
5. Fold in the shrimp and continue cooking for 5 minutes or until it's opaque.
6. Combine the pasta and shrimp together and top it off with the cheese to serve.

Slow Cooked Lemon Chicken

Serving Yields: 6
Nutritional Calorie Count: 336

Ingredients Needed:

- Bone-in chicken breast halves - 6 - 12 oz. each
- Dried oregano -1 tsp.
- Seasoned salt - .5 tsp.
- Pepper - .25 tsp.
- Butter - 2 tbsp.
- Water - .25 cup
- Fresh parsley - 2 tsp.
- Minced garlic - 2 cloves
- Lemon juice - 3 tbsp.
- Chicken bouillon granules - 1 tsp.
- Optional: Cooked hot rice
- Also Needed: 5-quart slow cooker & skillet

Preparation Instructions:

1. Remove the skin from chicken. Pat it dry with paper towels.
2. Combine the pepper, seasoned salt, and oregano; rub over the chicken.
3. Prepare a skillet using the medium heat setting, and add the butter.
4. Brown the chicken. Transfer into the cooker.
5. Pour the water over the chicken.
6. Secure the lid and set on the low setting for 5 to 6 hours.
7. Baste the chicken with the cooking juices. Add the minced parsley. Place the lid on the pot and cook for 15 to 30 minutes longer.
8. Serve with a portion of rice if desired.

Speedy Tilapia with Avocado & Red Onion

Serving Yields: 4
Nutritional Calorie Count: 200

Ingredients Needed:

- Extra-virgin olive oil - 1 tbsp.
- Sea salt .25 tsp.
- Fresh orange juice - 1 tbsp.
- Tilapia fillets - four 4 oz. . - more oblong than square
- Red onion - .25 cup
- Sliced avocado - 1
- Also Needed: 9-inch pie plate

Preparation Instructions:

1. Combine the salt, juice, and oil together. Add to the pie dish. Work with one fillet at a time. Place in the dish and turn to coat all sides.
2. Arrange the fillets in a wagon wheel shaped formation so that one of each of the fillets are in the center of the dish with the other end draped over the edge of the dish.
3. Place a tablespoon of the onion on top of each of the fillets and fold the end into the center. When done. you will have four folded fillets with the fold against the outer edge of the dish.
4. Cover the dish with plastic wrap. Leave one corner open to vent the steam.
   Place in the microwave on high for 3 minutes. It's done when the center can be easily flaked.
5. Top the fillets off with the avocado and serve.

Snacks for the Fall/Autumn

Honey Nut Granola

Serving Yields: 6
Nutritional Calorie Count: 337

Ingredients Needed:

- Regular rolled oats - 2.5 cups
- Coarsely chopped almonds - .33 cup
- Cinnamon - .5 tsp.
- Sea salt - .125 tsp.
- Chopped dried apricots - .5 cup
- Ground flaxseed - 2 tbsp.
- Honey - .25 cup
- Vanilla extract - 2 tsp.
- Extra-virgin olive oil - .25 cup

Preparation Instructions:

1. Warm up the oven to reach 325° Fahrenheit.
2. Place a layer of parchment paper onto a rimmed baking sheet.
3. In a large skillet, combine the cinnamon, salt, almonds, and the oats.
4. Use the medium-high temperature setting and toast for about 6 minutes, stirring often.
5. Stir the oil, honey, flaxseed, and the apricots. Cook in the microwave for one minute. You can also use a small saucepan over medium heat for about 3 minutes.
6. Add the vanilla into the honey mixture and pour the oats in the skillet.

7. Spread out on the pan. Bake for approximately 15 minutes.
8. Cool completely and break into small pieces. Store in the refrigerator for up to two weeks.

Honey Rosemary Almonds

Serving Yields: 6
Nutritional Calorie Count: 149

Ingredients Needed:

- Raw - whole - shelled almonds - 1 cup
- Minced fresh rosemary - 1 tbsp.
- Sea salt - .25 tsp.
- Honey - 1 tbsp.

Preparation Instructions:

1. Use the medium heat setting to warm a skillet. Toss in the rosemary, salt, and almonds.
2. Drizzle with the honey and continue cooking for 3 to 4 minutes.
3. Stir often until the almonds are well coated and starting to darken around the edges
4. Transfer to the countertop. Use a spatula to spread the almonds evenly onto a pan coated with a spritz of nonstick cooking oil spray.
5. Cool for 10 minutes and break the almonds apart right before serving.

Italian Vanilla Greek Yogurt Affogato

Serving Yields: 4
Nutritional Calorie Count: 270

Ingredients Needed:

- Vanilla Greek yogurt - 24 oz.
- Sugar - 2 tsp.
- Hot espresso - 4 Shots or 0.75 of a cup strong brewed coffee
- Chopped - unsalted pistachios - 4 tbsp.
- Dark chocolate chips or shavings - 4 tbsp.

Preparation Instructions:

1. Spoon the yogurt into four tall glasses.
2. Mix .5 teaspoon of sugar into each of the espresso shots.
3. Pour one shot of hot espresso or 1.5 oz. of coffee into each of the yogurt glasses.
4. Top each one off with the chocolate chips and pistachios before serving.

Kale Chips

Serving Yields: 4
Nutritional Calorie Count: 56

Ingredients Needed:

- Olive oil - 1 tbsp.
- Chili powder - .5 tsp.
- Fine sea salt - .25 tsp.
- Steamed kale - 2-inch pieces
- Also Needed: 2 baking sheets

Preparation Instructions:

1. Warm up the oven to reach 300° Fahrenheit.
2. Line each of the pans with parchment paper.
3. Rinse and dry the kale. Add to a bowl with the olive oil.
4. Spread the kale out on the baking sheets (single layered). Roast for 25 minutes.
5. Let them cool for 5 minutes before serving.

Spiced Sweet Roasted Red Pepper Hummus

Serving Yields: 8
Nutritional Calorie Count: 64

Ingredients Needed:

- Garbanzo beans - drained - 15 oz. can
- Lemon juice - 3 tbsp.
- Roasted red peppers - 1 - 4 oz. jar
- Tahini - 1.5 tbsp.
- Minced garlic - 1 clove
- Cayenne pepper - .5 tsp.
- Salt - .25 tsp.
- Ground cumin - .5 tsp.
- Chopped fresh parsley - 1 tbsp.

Preparation Instructions:

1. Prepare all of the fixings in a food processor or blender.
2. When fluffy and smooth; add to a serving dish for at least one hour. Return to the room temperature when it is time to serve.

Walnut & Date Smoothie

Serving Yields: 2
Nutritional Calorie Count: 385

Ingredients Needed:

- Pitted dates - 4
- Milk - .5 cup
- Plain Greek yogurt - 2 cups
- Walnuts - .5 cup
- Cinnamon - .5 tsp.
- Pure vanilla extract - .5 tsp.
- Ice cubes - 2-3

Preparation Instructions:

1. Combine all of the fixings together.
2. Pulse in the blender until smooth and creamy.
3. Serve in chilled glasses.

Chapter 8: Recipes for the Winter Months

Breakfast Favorites for Winter

Barley Porridge

Serving Yields: 4
Nutritional Calorie Count: 354

Ingredients Needed:

- Wheat berries - 1 cup
- Barley - 1 cup
- Unsweetened almond milk - 2 cups (+) more for serving
- Blueberries - .5 cup
- Pomegranate seeds - .5 cup
- Water - 2 cups
- Roasted and chopped hazelnuts - .5 cup
- Raw honey - .25 cup

Preparation Instructions:

1. Pour the almond milk, water, wheat berries, and barley into a saucepan using the medium-high heat setting.
2. Once boiling, reduce the heat to the low setting. Let it simmer for 25 minutes.
3. Stir often. When done, top each serving with the pomegranate seeds, a tablespoon of honey, the blueberries, and hazelnuts. Give it a splash of the almond milk. Serve.

Christmas Breakfast Sausage Casserole

Serving Yields: 8
Nutritional Calorie Count: 377

Ingredients Needed:

- Ground pork sausage - 1 lb.
- Mustard powder - 1 tsp.
- Salt - .5 tsp.
- Eggs - 4
- Milk - 2 cups
- White bread - 6 slices - toasted & cut into cubes
- Mild Cheddar cheese - shredded - 8 oz.
- Also Needed: 9 x 13-inch baking dish

Preparation Instructions:

1. Grease the baking pan.
2. Crumble the sausage into a skillet and prepare using the medium heat setting. Drain when done.
3. Whisk the eggs with the milk, salt, and mustard powder.
4. Stir in the cheese, bread cubes, and sausage.
5. Pour into the prepared baking dish and place a cover on top.
6. Chill for at least 8 hours or overnight for best results.
7. Warm up the oven to reach 350° Fahrenheit.
8. Bake for 45 to 60 minutes.
9. Remove the lid, and lower the temperature to 325° Fahrenheit. Bake for 30 minutes or until set.

Crustless Spinach Quiche

Serving Yields: 6
Nutritional Calorie Count: 309

Ingredients Needed:

- Vegetable oil - 1 tbsp.
- Chopped onion - 1
- Frozen chopped spinach - 1 (10 oz.) pkg.
- Eggs - 5
- Shredded Muenster cheese - 3 cups
- Salt - .25 tsp.
- Ground black pepper - .125 tsp.
- Also Needed: 9-inch pie pan

Preparation Instructions:

1. Thaw and drain the spinach.
2. Warm up the oven to reach 350° Fahrenheit. Lightly grease the baking pan with cooking oil spray.
3. Heat up a skillet using the med-high heat setting. Toss in the onions and sauté until softened. Fold in the spinach and cook until the moisture is absorbed.
4. Whisk the eggs with the salt, pepper, and cheese. Add the thawed spinach mixture. Stir well and scoop into the pan.
5. Bake about 30 minutes. Let cool for about 10 minutes before serving.

French Toast Delight

Serving Yields: 12
Nutritional Calorie Count: 123

Ingredients Needed:

- All-purpose flour - .25 cup
- Milk - 1 cup
- Salt - 1 pinch
- Eggs - 3
- Ground cinnamon - .5 tsp.
- Vanilla extract - 1 tsp.
- White sugar - 1 tbsp.
- Thick slices bread - 12

Preparation Instructions:

1. Measure the flour and add to a mixing bowl. Whisk in the sugar, milk, vanilla extract, cinnamon, eggs, and salt.
2. Warm up a frying pan or lightly oiled griddle using the medium heat setting.
3. Soak the bread in the mixture until fully saturated.
4. Prepare each side of the French toast until golden brown.
5. Serve hot.

Fruit Bulgur Breakfast Bowl

Serving Yields: 6
Nutritional Calorie Count: 301

Ingredients Needed:

- 2% milk - 2 cups
- Uncooked bulgur - 1.5 cups
- Water - 1 cup
- Cinnamon - .5 tsp.
- Frozen/fresh pitted dark sweet cherries - 2 cups
- Dried/fresh chopped figs - 8
- Chopped almonds - .5 cup

Preparation Instructions:

1. Combine the cinnamon, water, milk, and the bulgur.
2. Stir once and bring to a boil. Put a top on the pot and lower the heat to medium-low.
3. Simmer for ten minutes or until liquid is absorbed.
4. Extinguish the flame, but leave the pan on the stove and stir in the cherries (if frozen no need to thaw), almonds, and figs.
5. Stir well to thaw the cherries and hydrate the figs. Stir in the mint, and scoop into serving bowls.
6. If desired, serve with warm milk or serve it chilled.

Greek Yogurt Bowl With Peanut Butter & Bananas

Serving Yields: 4
Nutritional Calorie Count: 370

Ingredients Needed:

- Medium bananas - 2
- Flaxseed meal - .25 cup
- Nutmeg - 1 tsp.
- Vanilla flavored Greek yogurt - 4 cups
- Peanut butter - .25 cup

Preparation Instructions:

1. Prepare four serving bowls with the yogurt. Top it off banana slices.
2. Put the peanut butter in a heatproof dish in the microwave to melt for 30 to 40 seconds.
3. Drizzle 1 tbsp. of the melted peanut butter over the sliced bananas. Sprinkle with the nutmeg and flaxseed meal. Serve right away and enjoy.

Marinara Eggs with Parsley

Serving Yields: 6
Nutritional Calorie Count: 122

Ingredients Needed:

- Extra-virgin olive oil - 1 tbsp.
- Chopped medium onion - .5 of 1 or 1 cup
- Minced garlic - 2 cloves or 1 tsp.
- Diced tomatoes - undrained - no-salt-added - 2 - 14.5 oz. cans
- Large eggs - 6
- Chopped Italian fresh flat-leaf parsley - .5 cup
- Optional: Crusty Italian bread with grated parmesan or Romano cheese

Preparation Instructions:

1. Prepare a skillet using the med-high heat setting and pour in the oil.
2. Dice the onion and toss it into the pan to sauté for about 5 minutes. Stir occasionally and add the garlic; continue stirring for another minute.
3. Add tomatoes with the juices into the pan and let it cook until bubbling for 2 to 3 minutes.
4. Crack an egg into a coffee mug.
5. Once the tomatoes are boiling, lower the heat to medium.
6. Use the spoon to make 6 indentions in the tomato mixture.
7. Add the egg to one of the slots and continue until you've used all of the eggs.
8. Place a top on the pot. Cook for 6 to 7 minutes or until they are the way you like them.
9. Top with the parsley and serve with bread and grated cheese if desired.

Lunch Options for the Winter

Chicken & White Bean Soup

Serving Yields: 6
Nutritional Calorie Count: 248

Ingredients Needed:

- Cooked cannellini beans - 15 oz.
- Cooked shredded chicken - 4 cups
- Leeks- .25-inch rounds - 2
- Freshly chopped sage - 1 tbsp.
- Chicken broth - 28 oz.
- Olive oil - 2 tsp.
- Water - 2 cups

Preparation Instructions:

1. Add the oil to a large saucepan and warm it up using the medium-high heat setting.
2. Cook for 3 minutes after adding the leeks. Stir in the sage and continue cooking 30 more seconds.
3. Pour in the water and chicken broth. Turn the heat to high and let it boil. Cover the pan and add the chicken. Stir. Cook for 3 minutes and uncover the pan.
4. Ladle the soup into the bowls and serve.

Chicken Marrakesh

Serving Yields: 8
Nutritional Calorie Count: 290

Ingredients Needed:

- Skinless breast halves - 2 lb.
- Cooked chickpeas - 15 oz.
- Large carrots - 2
- Large sweet potatoes - 2
- Diced tomatoes - 14.5 oz.
- Minced garlic - 1 tsp.
- Medium white onion - 1
- Salt - 1 tsp.
- Turmeric - .5 tsp.
- Dried parsley - 1 tsp.
- Cinnamon - .25 tsp.
- Ground cumin - .5 tsp.
- Black pepper - .5 tsp.
- Suggested: 6-quart slow cooker

Preparation Instructions:

1. Lightly grease the slow cooker.
2. Slice the chicken into 2-inch pieces. Peel and dice the carrots, sweet potatoes, and white onions. Mince the garlic.
3. Stir or whisk the cumin, parsley, turmeric, black pepper, and salt together.
4. Add everything into the greased cooker.
5. Secure the lid on the cooker and set the timer for 4 to 5 hours. The chicken should be done throughout and the potatoes should be tender.
6. Serve immediately.

Cucumber Dill Greek Yogurt Salad

Serving Yields: 6
Nutritional Calorie Count: 49.6

Ingredients Needed:

- Large cucumbers - 4 sliced
- Dried dill - 1 tbsp.
- Garlic powder - .25 tsp.
- Salt - .5 tsp.
- Ground black pepper - .25 tsp.
- Sugar - .5 tsp.
- Apple cider vinegar - 1 tbsp.
- Greek yogurt - 4 tbsp.

Preparation Instructions:

1. Combine all of the fixings except for the cucumber in a mixing dish. Whisk until well combined.
2. Add the sliced cucumbers and toss well.
3. Chill the salad for about 10 minutes in the fridge before serving.

Dill Salmon Salad Wraps

Serving Yields: 6
Nutritional Calorie Count: 336

Ingredients Needed:

- Salmon fillet - 1 lb. cooked or 3 - 5-oz. cans
- Carrots - .5 cup - 1 carrot
- Celery - .5 cup - 1 stalk
- Fresh dill - 3 tbsp.
- Diced red onion - 3 tbsp.
- Capers - 2 tbsp.
- Extra-virgin olive oil - 1.5 tbsp.
- Aged balsamic vinegar - 1 tbsp.
- Freshly cracked black pepper - .5 tsp.
- Sea salt or kosher salt - .25 tsp.
- Whole wheat flatbread wraps or soft whole wheat tortillas - 4

Preparation Instructions:

1. Prep the veggies. Dice the carrots, celery, and red onion. Chop the fresh dill.
2. Combine the vinegar, pepper, salt, oil, capers, red onion, dill, celery, carrots, and salmon in a large mixing bowl. Mix well.
3. Divide the salmon salad into your chosen bread. Fold it up or wrap it, and serve.

Fried Rice With Spinach – Peppers & Artichokes

Serving Yields: 4
Nutritional Calorie Count: 244

Ingredients Needed:

- Cooked rice - 1.5 cups
- Frozen chopped spinach - 10 oz.
- Marinated artichoke hearts - 6 oz.
- Roasted red peppers - 4 oz.
- Minced garlic - .5 tsp.
- Crumbled feta cheese with herbs - .5 cup
- Olive oil - 2 tbsp.

Preparation Instructions:

1. Prepare the vegetables. Mince the garlic. Thaw and drain the frozen spinach. Drain and quarter the artichoke hearts. Drain and chop the roasted red peppers.
2. Use the medium temperature setting on the stovetop to warm up a skillet. Warm up the oil. Toss in the garlic to cook for 2 minutes.
3. Toss in the rice and continue cooking for about 2 minutes until well heated.
4. Fold in the spinach and continue cooking for 3 more minutes.
5. Add the red peppers and artichoke hearts. Simmer for 2 minutes.
6. Stir in the feta cheese and remove the pan from the burner.
7. Serve immediately.

Italian Tuna Sandwiches

Serving Yields: 4
Nutritional Calorie Count: 347

Ingredients Needed:

- Extra-virgin olive oil - 2 tbsp.
- Freshly squeezed lemon juice - 1 medium lemon - 3 tbsp.
- Minced garlic - 1 clove - .5 tsp.
- Freshly cracked black pepper - .5 tsp.
- Drained tuna - 2 - 5 oz. cans
- Sliced olives - black or green - 2.25 oz. or about .5 cup
- Celery (1 stalk) or freshly chopped fennel - .5 cup
- Whole grain crusty bread - 8 slices

Preparation Instructions:

1. Whisk the lemon juice, pepper, garlic, and oil.
2. Drain and fold in the tuna, fennel, and olives. Break the chunks of tuna apart with a fork and stir well to combine all of the fixings.
3. Divide over four slices of bread and put the tops on to serve. Let the sandwiches sit for at least five minutes so the filling can soak up the bread before serving.

Mediterranean Bean Salad

Serving Yields: 4
Nutritional Calorie Count: 329

Ingredients Needed:

- Drained garbanzo beans - 15.5 oz.
- Drained kidney beans - 15 oz.
- Lemon - 1 juiced and zested
- Chopped medium tomato - 1
- Salt - .5 tsp.
- Chopped red onion - .25 cup
- Chopped fresh parsley - .5 cup
- Rinsed and drained capers - 1 tsp.
- Extra-virgin olive oil - 3 tbsp.

Preparation Instructions:

1. Combine all the fixings in a large bowl.
2. Cover with plastic or a lid and place in the fridge for about 2 hours.
3. Stir occasionally before serving.

Dinner Specialties for the Winter

Beef Cacciatore

Serving Yields: 6
Nutritional Calorie Count: 510

Ingredients Needed:

- Steak of choice - 1 lb.
- Red bell peppers - 2 medium
- Orange bell pepper - 1 medium
- White onion - 1 medium
- Olive oil - .25 cup
- Tomato sauce - 1 cup
- Black pepper - .5 tsp.
- Salt - 1 tsp.

Preparation Instructions:

1. Slice the beef into thin slices. Chop the peppers and onions.
2. Prepare until pureed a large pot using the medium heat setting. When hot, add the oil and beef. Cook for 7 to 10 minutes.
3. Toss in the onion. Sauté for 1 additional minute or until it starts to soften.
4. Add the peppers and cook for two more minutes. Sprinkle with the salt and pepper. Pour in the tomato sauce.
5. Stir and remove from the heat.
6. Add to a food processor, but leave the meat in the pot. Pulse for 1 minute until pureed.
7. Add the sauce back into the pot and mix well. Simmer five minutes using medium heat or until heated well. Stir constantly.
8. Serve with cooked pasta.

Beef With Artichokes – Slow Cooker

Serving Yields: 6
Nutritional Calorie Count: 416

Ingredients Needed:

- Stewing beef - 2 lb.
- Artichoke hearts - 14 oz.
- Kalamata olives - .5 cup
- Diced tomatoes - 14.5 oz. can
- Minced garlic - 2 tsp.
- Beef broth - 32 fluid oz.
- Ground cumin - .5 tsp.
- Dried oregano - 1 tsp.
- Dried parsley - 1 tsp.
- Dried basil - 1 tsp.
- Bay leaf - 1
- Grapeseed oil - 1 tbsp.
- Tomato sauce - 15 oz.
- Also Needed: 6-quart slow cooker

Preparation Instructions:

1. Drain and chop the artichokes into halves. Dice the garlic. Remove the pit from the olives and chop.
2. Add oil to a large pot using the medium-high heat setting.
3. Once it's hot, add the beef, and cook for about 2 minutes on each side.
4. Transfer the beef into the cooker and add the rest of the fixings.
5. Secure the lid and set the timer for 7 hours using the low heat setting.

Mediterranean Pork Chops

Serving Yields: 4
Nutritional Calorie Count: 161

Ingredients Needed:

- Boneless pork loin chops - 4 - .5-inch cut
- Salt - .25 tsp.
- Dried rosemary - 1 tsp.
- Ground black pepper - .25 tsp.
- Minced garlic - 1.5 tsp.

Preparation Instructions:

1. Warm up the oven to 425° Fahrenheit.
2. Season the chops with the salt and pepper. Set to the side.
3. Whisk the rosemary and garlic together. Rub into the pork chops.
4. Prepare a roasting pan with a layer of aluminum foil. Arrange the chops in it. Place in the oven.
5. Lower the temperature to 350° Fahrenheit and roast for 25 minutes.
6. Serve right away.

Nicoise-Style Tuna Salad with Olives & White Beans

Serving Yields: 4
Nutritional Calorie Count: 548

Ingredients Needed:

- Green beans - .75 lb.
- Solid white albacore tuna - 12 oz. can
- Great Northern beans - 16 oz. can
- Sliced black olives - 2.25 oz.
- Thinly sliced medium red onion - .25 of 1
- Large hard-cooked eggs - 4
- Dried oregano - 1 tsp.
- Extra-virgin olive oil - 6 tbsp.
- Lemon juice - 3 tbsp.
- Ground black pepper and salt - to taste
- Finely grated lemon zest - .5 tsp.
- Water - .33 cup

Preparation Instructions:

1. Drain the can of tuna, Great Northern beans, and black olives. Trim and snap the green beans into halves. Thinly slice the red onion. Cook and peel the eggs until hard boiled.
2. Pour the water and salt into a skillet and add the beans.
3. Place a top on the pot and turn the heat to high. Bring to a boil.
4. Once the beans are cooking, set a timer for 5 minutes. Immediately, drain and add the beans to a cookie sheet with a raised edge on paper towels to cool.
5. Combine the onion, olives, white beans, and drained tuna. Mix together with the zest, lemon juice, oil, and oregano.
6. Pour the mixture over the salad and gently toss.

7. Adjust the seasonings to your liking. Portion the tuna-bean salad with the green beans and eggs to serve.

Slow Cooked Roasted Turkey Breast

Serving Yields: 8
Nutritional Calorie Count: 333

Ingredients Needed:

- Boneless turkey breast - trimmed - 4 lb.
- Chicken broth - divided - .5 cup
- Fresh lemon juice - 2 tbsp.
- Chopped onion - 2 cups
- Pitted kalamata olives - .5 cup
- Oil-packed sun-dried tomatoes - thinly sliced - .5 cup
- Greek seasoning - such as McCormick's - 1 tsp.
- Salt - .5 tsp.
- Black pepper - .25 tsp.
- All-purpose flour - 3 tbsp.

Preparation Instructions:

1. Arrange the turkey breast, salt, Greek seasoning, tomatoes, olives, onion, lemon juice, and 1/4 cup of the chicken broth into the slow cooker. Secure the lid set the timer for 7 hours on the low setting.
2. Combine the rest of the broth with the flour in a small mixing container. Whisk until smooth and stir into the slow cooker at the end of the 7-hour cooking time.
3. Cover and continue cooking on low for another 30 minutes before serving.

Spanish Moroccan Fish

Serving Yields: 12
Nutritional Calorie Count: 268

Ingredients Needed:

- Vegetable oil - 1 tbsp.
- Onion - 1
- Garlic - 1 clove
- Garbanzo beans - 1 can - 15 oz.
- Red bell peppers - 2
- Large carrot - 1
- Tomatoes - 3
- Olives - 4
- Fresh parsley - .25 cup
- Ground cumin - .25 cup
- Paprika - 3 tbsp.
- Chicken bouillon granules - 2 tbsp.
- Cayenne pepper - 1 tsp.
- Salt - to taste
- Tilapia fillets - 5 lb.

Preparation Instructions:

1. Finely chop the garlic, onion, tomatoes, olives, and parsley. Drain and rinse the garbanzo beans. Slice the carrots and bell peppers.
2. Warm up the oil in a skillet using the medium heat setting.
3. Stir in the onion and garlic. Sauté until softened or about 5 minutes.
4. Stir in the bell peppers, olives, tomatoes, carrots, and the beans.
5. Simmer for about 5 more minutes.
6. Sprinkle with the paprika, cumin, parsley, chicken bouillon, and the cayenne over the veggies.

7. Dust with the salt and stir the vegetables. Add fish. Pour in enough water to cover the fish.
8. Set the temperature to low. Cook until the fish are flaky or about 40 minutes.

Sweet Sausage Marsala

Serving Yields: 6
Nutritional Calorie Count: 509

Ingredients Needed:

- Italian sausage links - 1 lb.
- Medium red bell pepper - 1
- Medium green bell pepper - 1
- Tomatoes - 14.5 oz. can
- Peeled large onion - .5 of 1
- Minced garlic - .5 tsp.
- Dried oregano - .125 tsp.
- Black pepper - .125 tsp.
- Marsala wine - 1 tbsp.
- Water .33 cup
- Uncooked bow-tie pasta - 16 oz.

Preparation Instructions:

1. Slice the onion and green peppers. Dice the tomatoes or purchase them precut.
2. Prepare a large pan of boiling water - about half full. Add the pasta and simmer for about 8-10 minutes.
3. Meanwhile, add the sausage to a medium skillet and pour in the water. Set using the medium-high heat temperature. Put a top on the pot and simmer for 8 minutes.
4. When the pasta is done, drain into a colander and set to the side for now.
5. Drain the sausage and return to the skillet. Stir in the wine, garlic, onion, and peppers. Simmer about 5 minutes using the medium-high temperature setting or until done.

6. Empty in the tomatoes and sprinkle with the oregano and black pepper.
7. Add the pasta and continue stirring. Remove the pan from the heat and serve.

Snacks for the Winter

Banana Sour Cream Bread

Serving Yields: 32
Nutritional Calorie Count: 263

Ingredients Needed:

- White sugar - .25 cup
- Ground cinnamon - 1 tsp.
- Butter - .75
- White sugar - 3 cups
- Eggs - 3
- Very ripe bananas, mashed - 6
- Sour cream - 16 oz. container
- Vanilla extract - 2 tsp.
- Ground cinnamon - 2 tsp.
- Salt - .5 tsp.
- Baking soda - 3 tsp.
- All-purpose flour - 4.5 cups
- Chopped walnuts (optional) - 1 cup
- Also Needed: 4 - 7 x 3-inch loaf pans

Preparation Instructions:

1. Warm up the oven to reach 300°Fahrenheit. Grease the loaf pans.
2. Sift the sugar and one teaspoon of the cinnamon. Dust the pan with the mixture.
3. Cream the butter with the rest of the sugar. Mash the bananas with the eggs and combine with the cinnamon, vanilla, sour cream, salt, baking soda, and the flour. Toss in the nuts last.

4. Pour the mixture into the pans. Bake for 1 hour. Test for doneness with a toothpick in the center. It's done when it comes out clean.

Chia Greek Yogurt Pudding

Serving Yields: 4
Nutritional Calorie Count: 263

Ingredients Needed:

- Chia seeds - .66 cup
- Hulled hemp seeds - 2 tbsp.
- Ground flaxseeds - 2 tbsp.
- Unsweetened soy milk - 1 cup
- Cinnamon - 1 tsp.
- Honey - 1 tbsp.
- Vanilla extract - 1 tsp.
- Greek yogurt - 1 cup

Preparation Instructions:

1. Whisk the milk and yogurt together in a large mixing dish.
2. Stir in the vanilla, cinnamon, honey, flaxseed, and hemp seeds.
3. Lastly, add the chia seeds and stir just enough to mix.
4. Place it in a container and chill for at least 15 minutes.
5. Stir again and chill for another hour. Serve as desired.

Chocolate Avocado Pudding

Serving Yields: 4
Nutritional Calorie Count: 295.3

Ingredients Needed:

- Large chilled avocados - 2
- Unsweetened cocoa powder - .33 cup
- Maple syrup - .33 cup
- Unsweetened vanilla extract - 2 tsp.
- Chopped hazelnuts - 4 tbsp.
- Full-fat coconut milk - unsweetened - .5 cup

Preparation Instructions:

1. Cut the avocados in half and remove the seeds. Scoop out the flesh and transfer to the food processor.
2. Add the rest of the fixings except for the nuts. Blend for 1 to 2 minutes until creamy smooth.
3. Spoon into four serving dishes and top with the nuts to serve.

Italian Apple Olive Oil Cake

Serving Yields: 12
Nutritional Calorie Count: 294

Ingredients Needed:

- Gala apples - 2 large
- Orange juice - for soaking apples
- All-purpose flour - 3 cups
- Ground cinnamon - .5 tsp.
- Nutmeg - .5 tsp.
- Baking powder - 1 tsp.
- Baking soda - 1 tsp.
- Sugar - 1 cup
- Extra-virgin olive oil - 1 cup
- Large eggs - 2
- Gold raisins - .66 cup
- Confectioner's sugar - for dusting
- Also Needed: 9-inch baking pan

Preparation Instructions:

1. Peel and finely chop the apples. Drizzle the apples with just enough orange juice to prevent browning.
2. Soak the raisins in warm water for 15 minutes and drain well.
3. Sift the baking soda, baking powder, cinnamon, nutmeg, and flour. Set aside.
4. Pour the olive oil and sugar into the bowl of a stand mixer. Mix on the low setting for 2 minutes or until well combined.
5. Blend while running, break in the eggs one at a time, and continue mixing for 2 minutes. The mixture should increase in volume, it should be thick - not runny.
6. Combine all of the ingredients well. Begin by making a well in the center of the flour mixture and add in the

olive and sugar mixture.
7. Remove the apples of any excess of juice and drain the raisins that have been soaking. Add them together with the batter, mixing well.
8. Prepare the baking pan with parchment paper. Spoon the batter into the pan and level it with the back of a wooden spoon.
9. Bake for 45 minutes at a 350° Fahrenheit.
10. When ready, remove the cake from the parchment paper and transfer into a serving dish. Dust with the confectioner's sugar. Warm up dark honey to garnish the top.

Maple Vanilla Baked Pears

Serving Yields: 4
Nutritional Calorie Count: 103.9

Ingredients Needed:

- Pears - 4
- Maple syrup - .5 cup
- Cinnamon - .25 tsp.
- Unsweetened vanilla extract - 1 tsp.
- For the Topping: Greek yogurt

Preparation Instructions:

1. Warm up the oven to reach 375° Fahrenheit.
2. Slice each of the pears into halves. Cut off a small sliver on the underneath side so it will lay flat.
3. Remove the seeds from the core and place on a baking sheet with the face side up and sprinkle with the cinnamon.
4. Whisk the syrup and vanilla. Drizzle over the pears. Save 2 tablespoons for the garnishing.
5. Place in the oven and bake for 25 minutes or until softened.
6. When done, place in the serving dishes and drizzle with the rest of the maple syrup mixture.
7. Serve with a dollop of yogurt.

Mediterranean Flatbread

Serving Yields: 6
Nutritional Calorie Count: 450

Ingredients Needed:

- Olive oil - 1 tbsp.
- Cooked cannellini beans - .66 cup
- Marinated artichoke hearts - 4 oz.
- Baby spinach - 2 cups
- Sliced medium avocado - .5 of 1
- Freshly torn basil leaves - .25 cup
- Halved cherry tomatoes - .5 cup
- Small red onion - .25 sliced
- Sea salt - .25 tsp. or as needed
- Freshly cracked black pepper - .125 tsp.
- Almonds - .25 cup
- Water - 2 tbsp.
- Crumbled feta cheese - 2 oz.
- Pita bread - 3 pieces

Preparation Instructions:

1. Heat up the oven to reach 350° Fahrenheit.
2. Prepare the food processor and add the water, oil, beans, almonds, pepper, salt, basil, and spinach. Pulse for one minute until creamy.
3. Spread the pita bread out on a large baking sheet. Spread with the prepared bean pesto.
4. Top it off with the artichokes, tomatoes, onion, and the avocado. Sprinkle with cheese.
5. Place the bread into the oven and bake about 10 minutes until they're crispy.
6. When ready, slice each piece into 4 segments and serve.

Serving Yields: 24 cookies
Nutritional Calorie Count: 187

Ingredients Needed:

- Vanilla extract - 1 tbsp.
- Extra-virgin olive oil - 1 cup
- Golden brown sugar - .75 cup
- Granulated sugar - .75 cup
- Kosher salt - 1 tsp. (+) extra for garnish
- Large egg - 1
- All-purpose flour - 2 cups
- Baking soda - .5 tsp.
- Semi-sweet chocolate chips - 2 cups

Preparation Instructions:

1. Warm up the oven to 350° Fahrenheit. Prepare 2 cookie tins with a sheet of parchment paper. Set to the side.
2. Pour in the vanilla, granulated sugar, brown sugar, olive oil, and the one tsp. of salt into a mixing container. Blend until it's creamy.
3. Whisk and add the egg.
4. Work in the baking soda and flour. Mix well and fold in the chocolate chips.
5. Use about 2 tbsp. for each cookie. Arrange on the baking sheets leaving about two inches between each one. Lightly sprinkle each one with the kosher salt.
6. Place the baking tins in the oven until the cookies are golden brown along the edges or about ten minutes.
7. Cool on the baking sheet for about 5 minutes.

Chapter 9: Recipes for the Spring Months

Breakfast Favorites for the Spring

Artichoke Frittata

Serving Yields: 4
Nutritional Calorie Count: 199

Ingredients Needed:

- Large eggs - 8
- Grated Asiago cheese - .25 cup
- Freshly chopped basil - 1 tbsp.
- Fine sea salt - .25 tsp.
- Black pepper - .25 tsp.
- Freshly chopped oregano - 1 tbsp.
- Olive oil - 1 tsp.
- Water-packed artichoke hearts - 1 can
- Chopped tomato - 1
- Minced garlic - 1 tsp.

Preparation Instructions:

1. Quarter and drain the artichoke hearts. Mince the garlic and chop the tomatoes, oregano, and basil.
2. Heat up the oven using the broil function.
3. Whisk the salt, pepper, eggs, oregano, basil, and cheese.
4. Prepare an ovenproof skillet over the med-high heat setting and olive oil.
5. Sauté the garlic for 1 minute. Remove the garlic from the skillet and stir in the egg. Add the garlic back into the mixture and sprinkle with the artichoke hearts and tomato. Cook without stirring for 8 minutes. The center should be set.

6. Place your skillet in the oven to broil for 1 minute. The top should be lightly browned. Serve warm.

Greek Egg Frittata

Serving Yields: 6
Nutritional Calorie Count:107

Ingredients Needed:

- Eggs - 6
- Milk - .5 cup
- Diced tomatoes - .5 cup
- Spanish olives - .25 cup
- Kalamata olives - .25 cup
- Chopped spinach - 1 cup
- Salt - 1 tsp.
- Crumbled feta - .25 cup
- Pepper - .5 tsp.
- Oregano - 1 tsp.
- Also Needed: Quiche pan or 8-inch pie pan

Preparation Instructions:

1. Program the oven to 400°F. Grease the baking pan.
2. Whisk the milk and eggs. Add the remainder of the fixings. Stir well.
3. Bake until the eggs are set, usually about 15-20 minutes.

Greek Yogurt Breakfast Parfait with Roasted Grapes

Serving Yields: 4
Nutritional Calorie Count: 300

Ingredients Needed:

- Seedless grapes - 1.5 lbs. - 4 cups
- Extra virgin olive oil - 1 tbsp.
- 2% plain Greek yogurt - 2 cups
- Honey - 4 tsp.
- Chopped walnuts - .5 cup

Preparation Instructions:

1. Warm up the oven to reach 450° Fahrenheit with the pan inside.
2. Wash the grapes and discard the stems. Wipe with a towel and put in a bowl. Spritz with oil and toss to coat.
3. Bake for 20 to 23 minutes. They will look slightly shriveled. Stir about halfway through the cooking process.
4. Take the pan from the oven. Cool for five minutes.
5. Meanwhile, assemble the parfaits by adding the yogurt to the glass.
6. Once the grapes are cooled, garnish the yogurt with a teaspoon of honey, 2 tbsp. of the walnuts, and a portion of the grapes.

Greek Yogurt Pancakes

Serving Yields: 6
Nutritional Calorie Count: 258

Ingredients Needed:

- Blueberries - .5 cup
- All-purpose flour - 1.25 cups
- Salt - .25 tsp.
- Baking powder - 2 tsp.
- Sugar - .25 cup
- Baking soda - 1 tsp.
- Unsalted melted butter - 3 tbsp.
- Eggs - 3
- Greek yogurt - 1.5 cups
- Milk - .5 cup

Preparation Instructions:

1. Rinse the blueberries and drain.
2. Sift the flour, baking soda, sugar, baking powder, and salt in a dish.
3. In another container, add the milk, yogurt, and butter. Whisk well.
4. Gradually the egg mixture into the dry fixings. Let the mixture rest for about 20 minutes.
5. At that time, prepare a large skillet using the medium heat setting.
6. Add butter into the skillet to melt.
7. Pour in the pancake batter, cooking for about 2 to 3 minutes or until bubbly. Flip it over and continue cooking for 3 minutes or until browned.
8. When ready, place on a serving dish and garnish with a spoonful of yogurt and berries. Serve.

Mediterranean Egg – Pepper & Mushroom Cup

Serving Yields: 12
Nutritional Calorie Count: 67

Ingredients Needed:

- Chopped mushrooms - 1.5 cups
- Chopped roasted bell peppers - 1.5 cups
- Garlic powder - .5 tsp.
- Salt - .125 tsp.
- Black pepper - .25 tsp.
- Eggs - 10
- Olive oil - 2 tbsp.
- Coconut milk - .66 cup
- Freshly torn basil leaves - as desired
- Crumbled goat cheese - 2.5 tbsp.

Preparation Instructions:

1. Warm up the oven to reach 350° Fahrenheit.
2. Prepare the cups of a 12-count muffin tray with a spritz of olive oil and set aside. You can also use paper liners if you choose.
3. Crack the eggs into a bowl along with the milk, black pepper, salt, and garlic powder. Whisk well.
4. Add the pepper and mushrooms until well mixed. Divide evenly into each of the cups.
5. Bake for 25 minutes or until the muffins are set and browned.
6. When ready, remove the tray and let it cool for about 10 minutes.
7. Top the muffins with basil and goat cheese to serve.

Overnight Blueberry French Toast

Serving Yields: 10
Nutritional Calorie Count: 485

Ingredients Needed:

- Day-old bread - 12 slices
- Cream cheese - 2 (8 oz.) pkg.
- Fresh blueberries - 1 cup
- Eggs - 1 dozen
- Milk - 2 cups
- Vanilla extract - 1 tsp.
- Maple syrup - .33 cup
- White sugar - 1 cup
- Cornstarch - 2 tbsp.
- Water - 1 cup
- Fresh blueberries - 1 cup
- Butter - 1 tbsp.
- Also Needed: 9 x 13-inch baking dish

Preparation Instructions:

1. Cut the bread and cream cheese into 1-inch cubes.
2. Lightly grease a baking pan. Put half of the bread cubes into the dish and top with a layer of cream cheese cubes. Sprinkle with 1 cup of the berries and top of the remainder of the bread cubes.
3. Whisk the milk with the eggs, syrup, and vanilla extract. Empty over the bread cubes and refrigerate overnight with a plastic cover or lid over the container.
4. Transfer the dish to the countertop approximately 30 minutes before baking time.
5. Warm up the oven to reach 350° Fahrenheit.
6. Place the lid on the dish and bake for 30 minutes.

Remove the lid and continue to bake for 25 to 30 more minutes or until the surface is lightly browned.
7. Combine the water, cornstarch, and sugar in a medium saucepan. Stir constantly for 3-4 minutes.
8. Fold in the rest of the blueberries and reduce the heat. Simmer for 10 minutes until the berries start to burst. Stir in the butter and pour over the baked French toast.

Roasted Asparagus Prosciutto & Egg

Serving Yields: 4
Nutritional Calorie Count: 199

Ingredients Needed:

- Fresh asparagus - 1 bunch
- Minced prosciutto - 2 oz.
- Salt - .125 tsp.
- Ground black pepper - .25 tsp.
- Lemon - .5 of 1 - zest and juice
- Apple cider vinegar - 1 tsp.
- Olive oil - 2 tbsp. - divided
- Eggs - 4

Preparation Instructions:

1. Warm up the oven to reach 425° Fahrenheit.
2. Place the asparagus in a baking tray with 1 tbsp. of oil and set aside.
3. Warm up a medium skillet using the medium-low heat setting. Add the remainder of the oil when hot and place into the pan. Simmer 3 to 4 minutes until browned. Spoon this over the asparagus.
4. Sprinkle with the black pepper to coat and place the baking tray in the oven to cook for 10 minutes.
5. Remove the tray from the oven and toss the asparagus. Place back in the oven and continue cooking for 5 more minutes.
6. Prepare a pan over high heat. Once it's boiling, lower the heat to medium, and pour in the salt and vinegar.
7. Crack an egg into a measuring cup and gently add into the boiling water. Simmer for 4-6 minutes until it's firm, and the egg yolk has thickened - but not hard. Place on a paper-lined plate using a slotted spoon.
8. Continue with the other three eggs until done.

9. Once the asparagus is roasted, spritz with lemon juice and divide on to the four plates.
10. Top it off with the poached eggs and a sprinkle of lemon zest and black pepper before serving.

Lunch Options for the Spring

Chicken & Veggie Wraps

Serving Yields: 4
Nutritional Calorie Count: 278

Ingredients Needed:

- Plain Greek yogurt - .25 cup
- Chopped chicken - cooked - 2 cups
- Red bell pepper - .5 of 1
- English cucumber - .5 of 1
- Shredded carrots .5 cup
- Scallion - 1
- Fresh thyme - .5 tsp.
- Fresh lemon juice - 1 tbsp.
- Multigrain tortillas - 4
- Sea salt & black pepper - .25 tsp. each

Preparation Instructions:

1. Dice the cucumber, scallion, and bell pepper. Chop the chicken. Shred the carrot.
2. Mix each of the fixings into a large bowl.
3. Spoon the mixture into each of the tortillas.
4. Fold and serve.

Chickpea Salad

Serving Yields: 4
Nutritional Calorie Count: 163

Ingredients Needed:

- Cooked chickpeas - 15 oz.
- Diced Roma tomato - 1
- Diced green medium bell pepper - .5 of 1
- Fresh parsley - 1 tbsp.
- Small white onion - 1
- Minced garlic - .5 tsp.
- Lemon - 1 juiced

Preparation Instructions:

1. Chop the tomato, green pepper, and onion. Mince the garlic.
2. Combine each of the fixings into a salad bowl and toss well.
3. Cover the salad to chill for at least 15 minutes in the fridge.
4. Serve when ready.

Escarole with Garlic

Serving Yields: 4
Nutritional Calorie Count: 66

Ingredients Needed:

- Escarole - 1 head
- Salt - 1 tsp.
- Red pepper flakes - .125 tsp.
- Garlic - 1.5 tsp.
- Olive oil - 1.5 tbsp.

Preparation Instructions:

1. Tear the escarole leaves.
2. Use the medium heat setting on the stovetop to prepare a skillet.
3. Once it's hot, add the oil and garlic. Sauté one to two minutes until lightly browned.
4. Stir in the leaves and pepper flakes in batches. Season each batch with salt and toss well.
5. Continue cooking for about 5 minutes until the leaves have wilted. Serve immediately to enjoy at its best.

Goat Cheese Salad

Serving Yields: 4
Nutritional Calorie Count: 322

Ingredients Needed:

- Garlic - 1 clove head
- Fine sea salt - .125 tsp.
- Black pepper - .125 tsp.
- Freshly chopped basil - 2 tsp.
- Goat cheese - room temperature - 4 oz.
- Whole wheat bread - 8 slices
- Freshly shredded spinach - 2 cups
- Roasted bell peppers - cut into half and into strips - 2
- Olive oil - as needed

Preparation Instructions:

1. Warm up the oven to reach 350° Fahrenheit.
2. Remove the top from the garlic head. Once they are exposed, drizzle with olive oil before placing on the baking sheet.
3. Roast the garlic for 20 to 25 minutes until soft and fragrant. Set aside and let them cool.
4. Combine the salt, pepper, basil, one teaspoon of garlic, and the goat cheese to make a soft mixture.
5. Toast the bread and lightly spread with the goat cheese mixture. Top each slice off with a quarter of the roasted peppers and a heap of spinach. Put it together and serve.

Greek Shrimp Farro Bowl

Serving Yields: 2
Nutritional Calorie Count: 428

Ingredients Needed:

- Shrimp - 16
- Uncooked farro - 4 oz.
- Medium shallot - 1
- Persian cucumber - 1 medium
- Roma tomato - 1
- Parsley leaves - 2 tbsp.
- Black pepper - 1 tsp.
- Salt - 2.25 tsp.
- Oregano leaves - 1 tsp.

Preparation Instructions:

1. Do the prep. Peel and devein the shrimp. Slice the cucumber and dice the tomato. Peel and quarter the shallot. Chop the oregano leaves. Juice the lemon.
2. Add water to a small saucepan and use the high heat setting. Add .75 tsp. of the salt and bring to a boil.
3. Pour in the farro and cook for 15 minutes with a lid on the pan.
4. In a bowl, and the cucumber, tomato, shallots, mint, oil, cheese, and vinegar with .5 tsp. of the salt and .5 tsp. of the pepper. Toss well and set aside.
5. Drain the farro and set to the side for now.
6. Whisk .5 tsp. of the black pepper, one teaspoon of salt, and lemon juice in a large mixing bowl. Add the shrimp and oregano; toss well.
7. Warm up a large skillet using the medium-high heat setting. Pour in the oil. When hot, add the shrimp in a single layer and prepare for 2 minutes per side.

8. Divide the farro between two serving dishes and add the cucumber salad topped off with shrimp.
9. Serve immediately and enjoy.

Mediterranean Tuna Salad

Serving Yields: 4
Nutritional Calorie Count: 328

Ingredients Needed:

- Cooked tuna in chunks - 12 oz.
- Small potatoes - 1 lb.
- Pimento stuffed green olives - .5 cup
- Sugar - 1 tsp.
- Green beans -1 lb.
- Ground black pepper - .5 tsp.
- Lemon juice - 1 tbsp.
- Brown mustard - 1 tbsp.
- Olive oil - 3 tbsp.
- For Serving: Chopped parsley & lemon wedges

Preparation Instructions:

1. Place a pot of water on the stovetop using the medium-high heat setting.
2. Add the potatoes. When boiling, reduce the heat setting and simmer for 5 minutes with the top on the pot until the potatoes are tender.
3. In a blender, pour in the lemon juice, mustard, pepper, olives, and sugar.
4. Mix until smooth or about 1 to 2 minutes.
5. Drain potatoes and veins. Divide the mixture into four serving platters.
6. Top it off with the olive mixture, and serve with lemon wedges.

Pasta With Sausage & Escarole

Serving Yields: 4
Nutritional Calorie Count: 333

Ingredients Needed:

- Uncooked bow-tie pasta - 3 cups
- Crumbled turkey sausage - 8 oz.
- Chopped escarole - 8 cups
- Diced fire-roasted tomatoes - canned - 14.5 oz.
- Small white onion - 1
- Red pepper flakes - 1 tsp.
- Minced garlic - 2 tsp.
- Salt - .25 tsp.
- Chicken broth - .75 cup
- Grated parmesan cheese - .25 cup
- Olive oil - 1 tsp.

Preparation Instructions:

1. Mince the garlic. Peel and chop the white onion and crumble the sausage.
2. Prepare a large saucepan with water and a little bit of salt.
3. Add the pasta once the water is boiling. Cook for 8-10 minutes.
4. Place a skillet on the stove over the med-high heat. Pour in the oil. When hot, add the onion and sausage. Sauté for about 5 minutes.
5. Add the broth, garlic, and escarole. Simmer for five more minutes until the escarole is tender.
6. Shake in the red pepper flakes and tomatoes. Simmer one more minute and remove the pan from the burner.
7. Drain the pasta into a colander. Add the escrow and toss until coated well.
8. Sprinkle with cheese and serve.

Dinner Specialties for the Spring

Chicken Thighs with Artichokes & Sun-Dried Tomatoes

Serving Yields: 6
Nutritional Calorie Count: 169

Ingredients Needed:

- Boneless chicken thighs - 6
- Julienne cut sun-dried tomatoes - 4 oz.
- Salt - 1.5 tsp.
- Grilled artichoke hearts - 14.75 oz. can
- Artichoke hearts liquid - .33 cup
- Minced garlic - 2 tsp.
- Black pepper - .75 tsp.
- Fresh parsley - 3 tbsp.
- Dried oregano - .5 tbsp.
- Suggested: 6-quart slow cooker

Preparation Instructions:

1. Drain the artichoke hearts (reserving .33 cup) and dice the sun-dried tomatoes. Mince the garlic cloves.
2. Sprinkle the chicken with the oregano, salt, and pepper. Arrange in a single layer in the cooker.
3. Add artichoke hearts, tomatoes, and garlic. Pour in the extra 1/3 cup of artichoke liquid.
4. Secure the lid and set the timer for 6 hours using the high heat setting.
5. When ready to serve, garnish with parsley.

Greek Honey & Lemon Pork Chops

Serving Yields: 4
Nutritional Calorie Count: 257

Ingredients Needed:

- Pork rib chops - 4
- Salt - .5 tsp.
- Cayenne pepper - .25 tsp.
- Lemon juice - 2 tbsp.
- Freshly snipped mint - 1 tbsp.
- Honey - 2 tbsp.
- Shredded lemon peel - 2 tbsp.
- Olive oil - 1 tbsp.

Preparation Instructions:

1. Remove all fat from the pork chops. Snip fresh mint and shred the lemon peel.
2. Slice the chops into 1-inch thick chunks, and put into a large resealable plastic bag.
3. Whisk the rest of the fixings and pour over the pork. Seal the bag.
4. Rotate the bag a few times and let it marinate for about 4 hours.
5. When ready to cook, prepare the grill. Grease the grilling rack with oil. Preheat using the medium heat setting.
6. Arrange the chops on the grilling rack. Grill for 5 - 6 minutes on each side. The meat thermometer should reach 160° Fahrenheit.
7. Serve immediately.

Greek Salad Tacos

Serving Yields: 4
Nutritional Calorie Count: 466

Ingredients Needed:

- Grilled chicken - 2 cups
- Black olives - .5 cup
- Romaine lettuce - 4 cups
- Tomatoes - 1 cup
- Cucumbers - .75 cup
- Cilantro - .25 cup
- Feta cheese - 1 cup
- Greek dressing - .5 cup
- Cucumber & Dill Dip - 1 cup
- Flour tortillas - 8

Preparation Instructions:

1. Do the preparation. Grill the chicken to your liking. Shred the lettuce and slice the black olives. Dice the tomatoes, cucumbers, and cilantro. Crumble the feta cheese and set aside.
2. Combine all of the fixings except for the tortilla, dip, dressing, and cheese.
3. Warm up the tortilla. Fill with the salad. Garnish with the dip and feta cheese.
4. Serve right way.

Grilled Lamb Chops with Mint

Serving Yields: 6
Nutritional Calorie Count: 238

Ingredients Needed:

- Lamb chops - 2.33 lb.
- Sea salt - 1 tsp.
- Red pepper flakes - .25 tsp.
- Minced garlic - 1 tsp.
- Freshly chopped mint leaves -.5 cup olive (+) more to garnish
- Olive oil - .33 cup

Preparation Instructions:

1. Prepare the grill with a generous amount of oil. Preheat using the medium-high heat setting.
2. Whisk the olive oil with the mint, pepper flakes, and salt. Use the rub over the chops.
3. Brush the chops with the mint oil and place on the grilling rack.
4. Cook for 3 to 4 minutes per side and put on the platter to serve.
5. Brush the chops with the remainder of the mint oil and a sprinkle of the mint. Serve.

Grilled Salmon

Serving Yields: 4
Nutritional Calorie Count: 214

Ingredients Needed:

- Salmon fillets - approx. - 4 - 5 oz. each
- Green olives - 4
- Minced garlic - 1 tbsp.
- Black pepper - .5 tsp.
- Fresh parsley - 1 tbsp.
- Fresh basil - 4 tbsp.
- Lemon - 4 slices
- Olive oil - as needed
- Lemon juice - 2 tbsp.

Preparation Instructions:

1. Chop the green olives, basil, and parsley. Thinly slice the lemon.
2. Warm up with the broiler. Use the high heat setting and place the cooking rack approximately four inches away from the heat source.
3. Whisk the lemon juice, parsley, basil, and garlic.
4. Lightly brush the fish with the oil mixture and sprinkle with the black pepper. Top it off with the prepared garlic mixture and place under the broiler.
5. Broil for 3 to 4 minutes. Place the fillets on aluminum foil. Continue to cook using the medium-low heat setting for approximately four minutes. When done, the fish will be opaque. The thickest part on a meat thermometer should read 145° Fahrenheit.
6. Transfer the salmon to a plate to serve with lemon slices and olives.

Mussels With Olives & Potatoes

Serving Yields: 4
Nutritional Calorie Count: 345

Ingredients Needed:

- Scrubbed mussels - 2.25 lb.
- Large peeled potatoes - 2
- Diced tomatoes - 14.5 oz.
- Sliced white onion - 1 medium
- Pitted green olives - .66 cup
- Minced garlic - 2 tsp.
- Cayenne pepper - .125 tsp.
- Salt - 1.5 tsp.
- Paprika - .5 tsp.
- Chopped fresh parsley - .5 cup
- Allspice - .125 tsp.
- Olive oil - 2 tbsp.
- Water - 1 cup

Preparation Instructions:

1. Peel the potatoes and cut into 1-inch cubes. Add to a pot of water, covering the potatoes with ¼-inch of water. Cover with plastic wrap.
2. Place in the microwave for 6 minutes using the high heat setting.
3. Prepare a large pot using the medium-high heat setting. Pour in the oil. When hot, toss in the garlic and onion. Simmer for 6 minutes.
4. Drain the potatoes and add to the cooker. Sprinkle with the allspice, paprika, pepper, and salt.
5. Stir well and simmer for 2 to 3 minutes. Pour in the tomatoes and water. Stir to remove the delicious brown bits from the bottom of the cooker.

6. Lastly, add the parsley, olives, and mussels. Simmer for 5 more minutes with a lid on. Serve immediately.

Salmon With Warm Tomato – Olive Salad

Serving Yields: 4
Nutritional Calorie Count: 433

Ingredients Needed:

- Salmon fillets - 4 - approx. 4 oz. - 1.25-inches thick
- Celery - 1 cup
- Medium tomatoes - 2
- Fresh mint - .25 cup
- Kalamata olives - .5 cup
- Garlic - .5 tsp.
- Salt - 1 tsp.
- Honey - 1 tbsp.
- Red pepper flakes - .25 tsp.
- Olive oil - 5 tbsp. (+) More for brushing
- Apple cider vinegar - 1 tbsp. (+) 1 tsp.

Preparation Instructions:

1. Slice the tomatoes and celery into 1-inch pieces and mince the garlic. Chop the mint and the olives.
2. Warm up the oven using the broiler setting.
3. Whisk 2 tbsp. of the olive oil, 1 tsp. of vinegar, honey, red pepper flakes, and 1 tsp. of the salt. Brush onto the salmon.
4. Line the broiler pan with aluminum foil. Spritz the pan lightly with olive oil, and add the fillets with the skin side down.
5. Place in the oven to broil for 4 to 6 minutes until well done.
6. Meanwhile, make the tomato salad. Mix .5 teaspoon of the salt with the garlic.
7. Prepare a small saucepan on the stovetop using the medium-high heat setting. Pour in the rest of the oil and add the garlic mixture with the olives and one

tablespoon of vinegar. Simmer for 3 minutes.
8. Prepare the serving dishes. Pour the bubbly mixture into the bowl. Add the mint, tomato, and celery. Dust with the rest of the salt and toss well.
9. When the salmon is done, serve with tomato salad.

Snacks for the Spring

Almond-Stuffed Dates

Serving Yields: 1
Nutritional Calorie Count: 149

Ingredients Needed:

- Whole almonds - 2 salted
- Pitted Medjool dates - 2
- Orange zest - .25 tsp.

Preparation Instructions:

1. Stuff each one of the dates with one of the almonds.
2. Prepare the zest and roll each of the prepared dates through the mixture.
3. Enjoy as a snack, anytime.

Date Wraps

Serving Yields: 16
Nutritional Calorie Count: 35

Ingredients Needed:

- Whole pitted dates - 16
- Thinly sliced prosciutto - 16 portions
- Black pepper - to taste

Preparation Instructions:

1. Wrap one of the prosciutto slices around each of the dates.
2. When done, serve with a shake of freshly cracked black pepper.

Mango Mousse

Serving Yields: 4
Nutritional Calorie Count: 358

Ingredients Needed:

- Medium ripe mangoes - 3
- Agave syrup - 3 tbsp.
- Coconut cream - 1.5 cup

Preparation Instructions:

1. Slice the mango to remove the stone.
2. Dice the flesh and place into a bowl. Mash them until smooth and puffy.
3. Add the coconut cream and whisk well. Whisk in the syrup. Spoon into the serving bowls.
4. Top off with a few chopped fruits and serve immediately.

Pistachio No-Bake Snack Bars

Serving Yields: 8 bars
Nutritional Calorie Count: 220

Ingredients Needed:

- Pitted dates - 20
- No-shell roasted & salted pistachios - 1.25 cups
- Rolled old fashioned oats - 1 cup
- Pistachio butter - 2 tbsp.
- Unsweetened applesauce - .25 cup
- Vanilla extract - 1 tsp.
- Also Needed: 8x8 baking dish

Preparation Instructions:

1. Use a food processor fitted with a metal blade.
2. Add the dates and process 30-45 seconds until pureed. Toss in the oats and pistachios. Pulse in 15-second intervals 2-3 times until a crumbly, coarse consistency achieved.
3. Place the applesauce, pistachio butter, and vanilla extract into the processor and pulse 20-30 seconds until dough is slightly sticky.
4. Line the pan with parchment paper.
5. Use a spatula to transfer the dough from the processor and pour into the pan. Press down firmly to evenly distribute the dough into the pan with another piece of parchment paper.
6. Lift the paper up and place evenly with the remaining 1/4 cup of no-shell pistachios onto the top of the dough.
7. Place the pan in the freezer with parchment paper on top and freeze for at least 1 hour before cutting.
8. Slice into 8 bars and store in an airtight container in the refrigerator for up to a week.

9. Note: To make pistachio butter, take 1 cup 'no-shell' pistachios and place in a food processor with 1 teaspoon vanilla extract. Process for 3-4 minutes, scraping down the sides as needed, until smooth.

Roasted Peaches & Blueberries

Serving Yields: 4
Nutritional Calorie Count: 45.7

Ingredients Needed:

- Peaches - 4
- Fresh blueberries - 1.5 cups
- Cinnamon - .33 tsp.
- Brown sugar - 3 tbsp.

Preparation Instructions:

1. Warm up the oven to reach 350° Fahrenheit.
2. Peel and slice the peaches. Arrange in a baking dish with the berries, a sprinkle of the cinnamon, and the sugar.
3. Use the broil setting. Let it cook for about 5 minutes and serve, or chill and serve.

Sautéed Apricots

Serving Yields: 4
Nutritional Calorie Count: 207

Ingredients Needed:

- Olive oil - 2 tbsp.
- Blanched almonds - 1 cup
- Sea salt - .5 tsp.
- Cinnamon - .125 tsp.
- Red pepper flakes - .125 tsp.
- Dried - chopped apricots - .5 cup

Preparation Instructions:

1. Prepare a frying pan using the high heat setting. Pour in the olive oil, almonds, and salt.
2. Sauté the almonds until golden which should take about 5 to 10 minutes. Stir frequently.
3. Spoon the almonds into a serving dish and add the chopped apricot, pepper flakes, and cinnamon.
4. Cool before serving.

Yogurt & Olive Oil Brownies

Serving Yields: 12
Nutritional Calorie Count: 150

Ingredients Needed:

- Olive oil - .25 cup
- Low-fat Greek yogurt - .25 cup
- Sugar - .75 cup
- Vanilla extract - 1 tsp.
- Eggs - 2
- Flour - .5 cup
- Cocoa powder - .33 cup (+) 1-2 tbsp. more if desired
- Baking powder - .25 tsp.
- Salt - .25 tsp.
- Chopped walnuts - .33 cup
- Also Needed: 9-inch square pan

Preparation Instructions:

1. Warm up the oven to 350° Fahrenheit.
2. Use a large spoon to combine the sugar, vanilla, and oil. Whisk the eggs and add to the mixture with the yogurt.
3. In another bowl, sift or whisk the flour, salt, cocoa powder, and baking powder. Stir in the olive oil mixture and the nuts and mix again.
4. Cover the pan with wax paper. Add the brownie mixture into the pan.
5. Bake for about 25 minutes. Let it cool thoroughly before removing the wax paper. Slice into squares.
6. Top it off with a portion of fresh berries of choice (add the extra calories.)

Conclusion

Staying busy is essential to combating food or drink cravings once you begin any new dieting technique. You need to remove the *craving* from your head, so you can break the hold it has on you. Try one or all of these suggestions. Organize your computer files. That could take a while if you are like most individuals.

Write in a journal about your health goals. Catch up on your favorite hobby or start one like drawing or painting to keep your hands and mind occupied. Look through some photo albums to break a smile. Call a friend and talk about anything that does not pertain to food or drinks. These are just a few of the things you can do to break the craving chain, but you get the idea.

Walk away with the knowledge learned and prepare a feast using your delicious new recipes and meal plan. Be the envy of the neighborhood when you provide a feast at the next neighborhood gathering. Show off your skills and be proud. You can also boast of how much better you feel using the Mediterranean diet plan.
Finally, if you found this book useful in any way, a review on Amazon is always appreciated!

Index for the Recipes

Chapter 6: Recipes for the Summer

Breakfast For Summer

- Broccoli & Cheese Omelet
- Egg White Scramble with Cherry Tomatoes & Spinach
- Peanut Butter & Banana Greek Yogurt Bowl
- Poached Eggs
- Prosciutto - Lettuce - Tomato & Avocado Sandwiches
- Scrambled Eggs with Spinach – Tomato & Feta
- Spinach Omelet

Lunch Options For The Summer

- Arugula Salad
- Cucumber Salad
- Feta Frittata
- Grecian Pasta Chicken Skillet
- Insalata Caprese II Salad
- Quinoa Fruit Salad
- Shrimp Orzo Salad

Dinner Specialties For The Summer

- Baked Salmon With Dill
- Feta Chicken Burgers
- Italian Chicken Skillet
- Lemon Chicken Skewers
- Rosemary Thyme Lamb Chops

- Summertime Mixed Spice Burgers
- Tomato Feta Salad

Snacks For The Summer
- Chilled Dark Chocolate Fruit Kebabs
- Fruit - Veggie & Cheese Board
- Garlic Garbanzo Bean Spread
- Honey Lime Fruit Salad
- Strawberry Greek Frozen Yogurt
- Watermelon Cubes

Smoothies
- Mango Pear Smoothie
- Strawberry Rhubarb Smoothie

Chapter 7: Recipes for the Fall & Autumn

Breakfast Favorites For Fall/Autumn
- Avocado & Egg Breakfast Sandwich
- Baked Ricotta & Pears
- Feta & Quinoa Egg Muffins
- Ham & Egg Cups
- Mashed Chickpea - Feta & Avocado Toast
- Pumpkin Pancakes
- Scrambled Eggs With Goat Cheese & Roasted Peppers

Lunch Options For Fall/Autumn
- Avocado & Tuna Tapas
- Cannellini Bean Lettuce Wraps

- Greek Lentil Soup
- Mushroom Risotto
- Roasted Tomato Pita Pizzas
- Stuffed Bell Peppers
- Stuffed Sweet Potatoes

Dinner Specialties For Fall/Autumn
- Braised Chicken & Artichoke Hearts
- Herb-Crusted Halibut
- Marinated Tuna Steak
- Pan Seared Salmon
- Penne with Shrimp
- Slow Cooked Lemon Chicken
- Speedy Tilapia With Avocado & Red Onion

Snacks For The Fall/Autumn
- Honey Nut Granola
- Honey Rosemary Almonds
- Italian Vanilla Greek Yogurt Affogato
- Kale Chips
- Spiced Sweet Roasted Red Pepper Hummus
- Walnut & Date Smoothie

Chapter 8: Recipes For The Winter Months
Breakfast Favorites For Winter
- Barley Porridge
- Christmas Breakfast Sausage Casserole

- Crustless Spinach Quiche
- French Toast Delight
- Fruit Bulgur Breakfast Bowl
- Greek Yogurt Bowl With Peanut Butter & Bananas
- Marinara Eggs With Parsley

Lunch Options For The Winter

- Chicken & White Bean Soup
- Chicken Marrakesh
- Cucumber Dill Greek Yogurt Salad
- Dill Salmon Salad Wraps
- Fried Rice With Spinach - Peppers & Artichokes
- Italian Tuna Sandwiches
- Mediterranean Bean Salad

Dinner Specialties For The Winter

- Beef Cacciatore
- Beef With Artichokes - Slow Cooker
- Mediterranean Pork Chops
- Nicoise-Style Tuna Salad With Olives & White Beans
- Slow Cooked Roasted Turkey Breast
- Spanish Moroccan Fish
- Sweet Sausage Marsala

Snacks For The Winter:

- Banana Sour Cream Bread
- Chia Greek Yogurt Pudding
- Chocolate Avocado Pudding
- Italian Apple Olive Oil Cake
- Maple Vanilla Baked Pears
- Mediterranean Flatbread
- Olive Oil Chocolate Chip Cookies

Chapter 9: Recipes For Spring
Breakfast Favorites For the Spring
- Artichoke Frittata
- Greek Egg Frittata
- Greek Yogurt Breakfast Parfait with Roasted Grapes
- Greek Yogurt Pancakes
- Mediterranean Egg - Pepper - & Mushroom Cup
- Overnight Blueberry French Toast
- Roasted Asparagus Prosciutto & Egg

Lunch Options For The Spring
- Chicken & Veggie Wraps
- Chickpea Salad
- Escarole with Garlic
- Goat Cheese Salad
- Greek Shrimp Farro Bowl
- Mediterranean Tuna Salad
- Pasta With Sausage & Escarole

Dinner Specialties For The Spring
- Chicken Thighs With Artichokes & Sun-Dried Tomatoes
- Greek Honey & Lemon Pork Chops
- Greek Salad Tacos
- Grilled Lamb Chops With Mint
- Grilled Salmon
- Mussels With Olives & Potatoes
- Salmon With Warm Tomato-Olive Salad

Snacks For The Spring
- Almond-Stuffed Dates
- Date Wraps
- Mango Mousse
- Pistachio No-Bake Snack Bars
- Roasted Peaches & Blueberries
- Sautéed Apricots
- Yogurt & Olive Oil Brownies

The Mediterranean Diet for Beginners:

The Complete guide for beginners, Mediterranean diet healthy Cookbook Recipes for Reser your metabolism, Plant, Practical Guide with 7 Simple Rules for Weight Loss and burn fat, Tips and paradox.

Table Of Contents

Introduction 184

Chapter 1: Understanding the Mediterranean Diet 187

Chapter 2: Benefits of the Mediterranean Diet 193

Chapter 3: Disadvantages of the Mediterranean Diet 204

Chapter 4: Being Keen on a Mediterranean Diet 208

Chapter 5: Mindset for Success on the Mediterranean Diet 222

Chapter 6: 14 Day Sample Meal Plan 227

Chapter 7: Mediterranean Diet Breakfast Recipes 255

Chapter 8: Mediterranean Diet Lunch Recipes 261

Chapter 9: Mediterranean Diet Dinner Recipes 269

Conclusion 280

Introduction

If you've downloaded this book, then you have probably heard about the very popular Mediterranean diet that has become a sensation. It has risen to the spot of #1 on lists of recommended diets because of its ease and flexibility to follow, but also because of the results it produces! The Mediterranean diet can help you achieve your primary goal of losing weight, but the overall benefits it produces can improve your quality of life and extend longevity.

The research and inspiration for this diet and lifestyle came from American scientist Ancel Keys, known as the "father of nutritional science." In his study of populations around the world, he noticed that less affluent people in the Mediterranean region lived longer and had fewer factors of heart disease than the richest people in New York City! With this information, he began a detailed study of diets around the world and how people's health was linked to their overall health and lifespan. Through his studies, he found the people in the Mediterranean region had the best overall health due to a mostly plant-based diet with good fats coming from olive oil, and nuts. Instead of a diet full of red meat, the Mediterranean diet focused on lean protein sources like fish, seafood, beans, and legumes.

Keys' study and subsequent studies have proven that the Mediterranean diet is the best method of losing weight and keeping excess weight off, but also improving overall health factors that can improve your quality of life. Switching to the Mediterranean diet can reduce your cholesterol, lower your blood pressure, keep your cognitive functioning more mentally alert, and protect against neurodegenerative diseases like Alzheimer's or Parkinson's. Even little changes like clearer skin and more energy can make a big difference when it comes to your health! With these changes, people have recognized the Mediterranean diet for what it is - a lifestyle change that can truly enhance and extend the span of your life.

What makes this diet so easy and flexible to follow? People love incorporating a Mediterranean diet lifestyle because of how user-friendly it is! There are no counting calories, decreasing your portion sizes, or counting your intake of macronutrients diligently all day. It's about learning what the diet entails and making those choices to fill your pantry and fridge with fresh, healthy ingredients that will promote better health. You will be cutting out the unhealthy things like processed foods, artificial sugars, refined grains, and soda from your diet which are known to cause blood sugar spikes and excess weight gains. Instead, you'll be shopping for ingredients rich in vitamins, minerals, good fats, and antioxidants that will improve your health! With a menu allowing whole grains, fish, seafood, fruit, vegetables, and even a glass of wine a day, the Mediterranean diet allows for such variety that you can't get sick of it! This is part of what it makes it such a great lifestyle choice for people to switch to and commit to dieting and eating healthy. Unlike other diets, it does not deprive you of the tasty things you would love to taste once in a while. It basically teaches you how to make the right choices by eating the right kinds of food that will not leave your palate craving for a tastier meal.

Along with the healthy diet full of lean protein and healthy greens, the Mediterranean diet encourages the addition of physical exercise. The people of the Mediterranean naturally incorporated physical activity into their day, whether it was walking, hiking, boating, or swimming. Working out at the gym will not be an everyday routine, but the idea is to become more physically active so you are able to burn calories and keep your body in its best shape. Exercise has so many benefits for our bodies so you're simply adding that along with the healthy diet you are committing to follow!

Any time you make changes to your diet or lifestyle, it's important you first speak to your physician about your desire for better health and what you're hoping to gain from this new diet. The Mediterranean diet can be beneficial for many people, but your individual health history matters. If you should not be consuming alcohol, or you have severe health concerns or take medication throughout the day, it's important you speak to your doctor about what adjustments you can make and if this diet is right for you.

With this book, we are here to teach you about the many detailed aspects of the Mediterranean diet including its history, health benefits, disadvantages, as well as how you can follow this lifestyle to lose excess weight! With tips to get started and ensure your success, as well as a 14-day beginner's meal plan along with other easy recipes for breakfast, lunch, and dinner, you are informed and able to make the conscious decision to improve your health today! We wish you the best success!

Chapter 1: Understanding the Mediterranean Diet

The general consensus has become that the Mediterranean diet is the healthiest and most preferred plan to help you lose weight and improve your overall health. When compared to many other diets that are making the rounds, people have found the Mediterranean diet very appealing its category of food to eat and the easy way it can be implemented into your daily life. There's no need to count calories or macronutrients which people find refreshing when it comes to living by the Mediterranean lifestyle and making it a part of their healthy diet. This diet focuses on a healthy variety of fresh fruits, vegetables, seafood, and fish. It forces us to break away from all the red meat we would commonly eat because of the dangerous health risks that come with it. By knowing exactly what you can and cannot eat, it makes it very easy to plan your meals without having to weigh food portions or count calories every meal.

The History of the Mediterranean Diet

Just like it sounds, the Mediterranean diet comes from the dietary traditions of the people of the Mediterranean isle region such as the Romans and Greeks. The people of these regions had a rich diet full of fruits, bread, wine, olive oil, nuts, and seafood. Despite the fatty elements in their diet, the people of this region tended to live longer and overall healthy lives with relatively less cardiovascular heart issues. This phenomenon was noticed by American scientist Ancel Keys in the 1950s.

Keys was an academic researcher at the University of Minnesota in the 1950s who researched healthy eating habits and how to reverse the decline in American cardiovascular health. He found in his research that poor people in the Mediterranean region of the world were healthier compared to the rich American population which had seen a recent rise in cardiovascular heart issues and obesity. Compared to wealthy New Yorkers, the lower class in the Mediterranean lived well into their 90s and tended to be physically active in their senior years. Keys and his team of scientists decided to travel the world and study the link between the region's diet and the health of the people who lived there. In 1957, he traveled and studied the lifestyles, nutrition, exercise, and diet of the United States, Italy, Holland, Greece, Japan, Finland, and Yugoslavia. Twenty years later, he published his findings in a landmark study called "The Seven Countries Study." It evaluated the diets and lifestyles of these regions and was one of the first studies to notice the link between cardiovascular disease and diet.

Keys' research found that the dietary choices of the people from the Mediterranean region allowed them to live a longer lifespan and one that kept them more physically active compared to other world populations. The people of Greece, in particular, ate a diet that consisted of healthy fats like seafood, nuts, olive oil, and fatty fish. Despite the amount of fat in these sources, their cardiovascular health stayed consistent without the risk factors for a heart attack or stroke. His study became a guideline for the United States to set its own nutritional standards, and he became known as the father of nutritional science.

With Keys' work leading the way, further research and clinical trials have been conducted on the Mediterranean diet which gives evidence for its health-improving properties. Not only will you lose weight, but you could lower your LDL "bad" cholesterol, lower your blood pressure, and decrease and stabilize blood sugar levels. With a decrease in these signs of cardiovascular heart disease, you can greatly reduce your risk of suffering from heart attack, stroke, or premature death.

It's important to point out that the Mediterranean diet cannot alone bring about these changes to someone's health. It will depend on a variety of other factors in their lifestyle such as genetics, physical exercise, smoking, obesity, drug use, etc. Part of the combination of the Mediterranean diet is incorporating physical exercise into your life. That's how it goes from the Mediterranean "diet" to a Mediterranean "lifestyle" that truly mimics the people of that region. The people of Greece tend to live an active lifestyle with some sort of daily physical activity they partake in. Whether that is walking, sailing, rowing, swimming, or hiking, coupling that physical exercise that with a healthy plant-based diet is what can bring about the beneficial health results. In our current environment, physical activity could mean a session at the gym or even just a walk around the block. It doesn't have to highly intensive, but the important part is incorporating some sort of physical activity in your day, so you can truly gain the benefits of following this diet.

Before we begin listing a rudimentary list of what you can and cannot eat, it's important to highlight that the Mediterranean region consists of many countries with their own unique dietary choices. With this diversity comes many varieties of recipes that you can incorporate into your dishes as long as you are still following the healthy tenets of the Mediterranean diet. This gives a basic outline of which foods you should include on your shopping list and then you can look for recipes from there! What does the basic Mediterranean diet look like?

- Your diet should consist heavily of whole grain bread, extra virgin olive oil, fresh fruits and vegetables, herbs and spices, nuts and seeds, fish and seafood

- You should moderately eat: poultry, cheese, egg, yogurt

- You should try to rarely eat: red meat and organ meat

- You should avoid the following: processed snacks, refined oils (canola oil or vegetable oil), refined grains (white bread), sugary drinks (juice, soda), processed meats (hot dogs, sausages, bacon), trans fats

- You should drink: water, wine

The Science behind the Mediterranean Diet

Most of the benefits of this form of diet come from a large number of plant foods associated with the diet. By incorporating a large number of fresh fruits and fresh vegetables in your diet, you are getting a high number of antioxidants and free radicals which are helpful for your body's cellular system and metabolism. The high intake of vitamins, minerals, and fiber you're getting from these plant sources can lower your risk of diabetes, constipation and bowel issues, and heart disease.

Since we've mentioned the Mediterranean diet's intake of healthy fats, it's important to go over why these are healthier for the body. Most of the fat is monounsaturated such as the fat you get from olive oil. This fat, found in nuts, seeds, and oil, tends to be healthier for the body compared to the saturated fat that is found in meat and poultry. A high amount of saturated fat is what tends to wreak havoc on the body's cholesterol and blood pressure.

By staying low in red meat intake, the Mediterranean diet harnesses protein sources from fish and seafood which are healthier for the body. They are high in omega 3 fatty acids. The research regarding omega 3 fatty acids is recent, covering the last 20 to 30 years, but it's shown to be an essential element for vision and brain health, as well as fetal health if a woman is pregnant. Adults are advised to consume at least 250 to 500 milligrams of fatty acids a day. Since most of us don't eat fish every day, you can get in the form of a fish oil supplement. With the Mediterranean diet, that won't be as necessary. The people of the Mediterranean had easy access to fishing and considered fresh fish and seafood a staple in their diet. Not only are there so many varieties, but it also is much healthier for you than having red meat many times a week which tends to raise your cholesterol and clog your arteries. You can still have red meat on this diet, but you should try to consume it more rarely and be aware of your portion sizes. And if you do have red meat, you want to ensure that you are also having healthy vegetables or whole grains along with it.

Along with food, it's important to note that drinking alcohol in moderation is a big part of the Mediterranean diet. Recent studies in the last decade have shown that moderate consumption of red wine could considerably lessen the risk of heart related diseases, gallstones, and diabetes (Type 2). It's believed that red wine contains a component called resveratrol which has health benefits in animals and humans. With this consumption, it's important to note that it is to be moderate, about a glass a day for women, and 2 for men. But with it can come health dangers for pregnant women or birth defects in babies. Many declare alcohol consumption as optional in the diet because some people may be restricted due to health or religious reasons.

We can't speak about the science behind the Mediterranean diet without speaking in length about extra virgin olive oil. With the abundance of olives in the Mediterranean region, olive oil is essential for all their cooking needs. That includes baking, seasoning, frying, and as a fat element in salad vinaigrettes. But when it comes to olive oil, the best oil will be labeled as "extra virgin" because it is the most unprocessed version of olive oil, so the purest that is available. There are many components in extra virgin olive oil that make it such a healthy substance. It contains a high amount of vitamin E which has anti-inflammatory properties for the body. It also has a high amount of phenol substances which contains similar health properties. Oleic acid is another property that is healthy for the heart. It's present in significant amounts in olive oil as compared to other oil types. When it comes to the properties of olive oil, it's taken very seriously by the culinary community. There's an International Olive Council that tests the levels of phenol and acidity in different brands of olive oil to ensure they qualify for the label of "extra virgin". The rule when it comes to olive oil is to go with the old saying "quality over quantity." Most nutritionists will say that consuming 4 to 5 tbsp of olive oil a day should be enough for all your cooking needs. That includes salad dressings, pan frying, baking, or seasoning your food. Olive oil should be kept away from direct sunlight and heat to avoid degradation of the oil.

When we see all these qualities of the Mediterranean diet and how they play out for the body, it's easy to see how this diet can help you improve your health. By including exercise in your routine, you are also gaining the possibility of better health and strengthening your heart and losing more weight. Along with the health benefits possible, the ease of the

Mediterranean diet appeals to many people. No counting calories, no measuring food portions, or keeping track of your daily macronutrients. With this flexibility and simply knowing the right foods to eat and avoid, the Mediterranean can be a very easy lifestyle to follow if you are hoping to improve your health.

Chapter 2: Benefits of the Mediterranean Diet

We've briefly discussed some of the Mediterranean lifestyle's health benefits and how it has become so successful for so many people. It has more benefits than just losing any extra weight! You can improve many health conditions like Type 2 diabetes or heart disease, and even help improve other facets of your health like acne, mental acuity, and hopefully extend the overall longevity of your lifespan. These aren't just people's experiences with the diet, but scientific research that has been conducted to find what the diet's benefits are.

What are some of the astounding health benefits possible on the Mediterranean diet? Here are some possibilities of how you could improve your health.

Losing weight and keeping it off! To many people, one of the best and appealing benefits of the Mediterranean diet is that you are able to lose weight by making healthier eating decisions. You do not have to starve yourself or cut your food portions, but by naturally shifting to more healthier foods, you can lose weight and keep that weight off. It's all about which foods you are eating to gain your nutrients. For example, you're staying away from red meat and relying on things like fish, legumes, and seafood as your sources of protein. You're also eating fresh fruits and vegetables which are packed with essential vitamins, minerals, and fiber that keep you full in between meals. You've also cut out the unhealthy items from your diet like sugar, processed foods, and refined bread. Some people may just start the Mediterranean diet to lose weight, so this may be the first goal they reach before they learn they can achieve many others!

Keeps your heart healthy and reduces risk factors of cardiovascular heart disease. As we mentioned in the previous chapter, there are many factors of the Mediterranean diet that improve heart health such as the addition of olive oil and wine. Olive oil is high in alpha-linolenic acid (ALA) which has been found to decrease the risk of cardiac or premature death by almost 30%. Compared to other oils like sunflower oil or vegetable oil, only olive oil has been found to significantly lower blood pressure. With a healthier diet focused on good fats, the Mediterranean diet can also maintain the HDL cholesterol in the body, the "good" cholesterol, and decrease the LDL "bad" cholesterol. Not only that, but it also reduces the level of unhealthy fatty triglycerides in the blood. A high level of these has been linked to an increased risk of stroke or sudden cardiac death. With the improvement of these risk factors, the body can have better blood flow and fewer plaque build-ups which keeps the arteries open and blood steadily pumping throughout the body. A study found that when obese men followed the Mediterranean diet, they had better blood flow compared to when they ate junk food and their arteries did not dilate.

Improves the longevity of your life. We have no guarantee of our future, but the research shows that the Mediterranean lifestyle may have the ability to increase your life span. A famous study called the Lyon Diet Heart Study followed patients who had suffered from heart attacks between 1988 and 1992. They were told to follow either a normal post-heart attack low-fat diet recommended by doctors at the time or the Mediterranean diet. Nearly 4 years after the study started, researchers found that the group who followed the Mediterranean diet had nearly 70% less risk of heart disease and 50% less risk of death than the followers of the low-fat diet. This longevity was also very much visible in the people of the Mediterranean that Ancel Keys first studied when he found the link between diet and quality of life. With all the benefits of the Mediterranean diet in improving your health, such as reducing the risk of cancer, heart disease, and neurodegenerative diseases, it's only logical that this will keep you healthy for longer. All by simply changing the types of food you're eating! Fresh fruits and vegetables tend to contain higher antioxidants which are great for strengthening your immune system and preventing disease.

Maintains eye vision and health. The Mediterranean diet includes a high amount of fish which means a high intake of omega 3 fatty acids. Unlike other triglycerides, these molecules play an important role in eye health. The American Academy of Ophthalmology ranks the Mediterranean diet as one of the best diets to protect and maintain eye health. Combined with the frequent servings of fish and seafood a week, there's also fresh fruits and vegetables that contain antioxidants. Studies show that having fish just once a week can decrease your chances of eye damage that can commonly occur in people over the age of 50, such as cataracts or cloudy vision. With the Mediterranean diet, you're having fish many times a week! Most of the general public doesn't have fish enough so they supplement with fish oil tablets, but with the Mediterranean diet, you'll be getting more than enough fatty acids. Fatty acids are also present in nuts and seeds which are a recommended snack in between meals.

Improves mental focus and cognitive functioning. Omega 3 fatty acids are composed of two parts: DHA and EPA. Along with vision health, as we mentioned above, they are also vital in brain development and functioning. They help preserve the health of brain cells and improve the communication between brain cells to allow for faster neural communication. As we get older, our brain is affected by natural signs of aging which can lead to the destruction of neural cells and neurodegenerative diseases like Alzheimer's, dementia, and Parkinson's. The omega 3 fatty acids of the Mediterranean diet are loaded with substances to protect the brain from premature aging and decline in functioning. Along with healthy fruits and vegetables, and removing processed foods and sugars from your diet, you can improve your memory recall, mental focus, and overall cognitive functioning.

Reduces your risk of having Type 2 diabetes. For people who have a family history of diabetes or who struggle with unstable blood sugar levels, this type of diabetes can feel imminent in their future. But the Mediterranean diet has been able to lessen the chances of acquiring diabetes (Type 2) because of its healthy eating patterns and allowing you to lose extra weight.

Studies have shown that patients can lose more weight following the Mediterranean diet than other low Carb or low-fat diet plans. This is a great way to reduce your risk of diabetes because extra weight is always a risk factor. Patients have seen improvements in their blood sugar levels and even been able to change their medication dosage, or quit it entirely! This diet encourages the consumption of fibrous foods like whole grains, beans, legumes, and fresh vegetables. When the body has enough fiber, it's able to slow digestion and make you feel full for a longer period of time. This minimizes the need for frequent snacking which is what can cause blood sugar spikes every time you eat. This means less insulin is produced. The Mediterranean diet doesn't follow a low carbohydrate philosophy, but it cuts foods that cause blood sugar spikes from your diet such as sugary snacks, refined grains, and soda.

Maintains bone density and overall agility of the body as you age. As we age, especially women, in particular, we lose bone density and muscle mass at an alarming speed. Recent research has found that when people who were over the age of 55 years followed the Mediterranean diet for a period of their life, they were able to have a higher level of bone mass and muscle mass compared to women who ate a diet consisting of red meat. It's important to note that for the Mediterranean diet to give these benefits, it has to be followed earlier than when menopause begins in most women. You cannot expect to only follow it for a few months and gain the benefits. It is a complete lifestyle change that you have to immerse yourself in so that you can feel confident in achieving the health successes further in your life. Whether it's the healthy fats that the Mediterranean diet brings to your diet, like the olive oil and fish, it protects the body and cushions the joints against aging, almost like lubrication.

Could help fight against cancer. There is a lot of research yet to cover in the area of cancer prevention, but some tentative research has labeled the Mediterranean diet has one of the best environments to combat cancer cells. A 2013 Italian research study found that the Mediterranean diet provided the highest levels of fiber, antioxidants, and omega 3 fatty acids compared to other diets. With the high intake of fruits, olive oil, fish, whole grains, vegetables, and wine, you're eating healthier, natural foods and avoiding the garbage of processed foods, trans fats, and sugar. It's important to note that diet only goes so far and this information is in the very beginning phases. You should always go for cancer screenings and annual health exams.

Can improve your digestive functioning and health. With a diet high in fiber from whole grains, fruits, and vegetables, it's no wonder the Mediterranean diet can help ease any digestive issues! Some diets make you constipated as they cut ingredients out of your diet, or reduce the intake of fiber drastically. With the Mediterranean diet focused on plant-based foods, it provides the body with healthy vitamins, minerals, and fiber. Studies have shown that those who consume predominantly meat had a lower variety of gut bacteria. Having more gut bacteria is essential for promoting digestive health and ensuring regular bowel movements to remove waste. Studies have shown that the more frequently your body expels waste, the less risk of developing colon cancer.

Could lower the risk of mental illnesses like depression and anxiety. Other areas where more research is necessary is in mental illnesses. Some research has linked depression, obsessive-compulsive disorder, and anxiety to high amounts of inflammation in the body. With the Mediterranean diet, you're eating high-quality foods that prevent inflammation. Fish and plant-based foods, in particular, have great anti-inflammatory properties, as well as the wine you're encouraged to drink in moderation.

Can clear acne breakouts and improve the look and health of your skin. Any dermatologist will tell you that sugar is bad for your skin and can cause pimples or acne breakouts. Not only that, it can destroy the natural collagen present under your skin which is what gives skin that youthful elasticity. The Mediterranean diet can help skin healthy two-fold: by having a diet rich in fruits and vegetables with natural antioxidants to keep the skin healthy, and by avoiding processed sugar that is found in baked goods and candy. The natural sugars found in fruit are not harmful to the body compared to refined sugar which can cause blood sugar spikes followed by skin irritations. Studies have found that when adult women who did not consume enough fish or fresh fruits and vegetables a week had nearly double the risk of having adult acne.

The Path to Weight Loss on the Mediterranean Diet

Often people will resort to desperate measures to lose weight, whether it's unhealthy diets, juice cleanses or fasting or intense exercising. With the Mediterranean diet, it's not meant to be a quick fix scenario - it's meant to be an entire lifestyle change. There have been many research studies that show losing weight is very possible on the Mediterranean diet compared to other low-fat diets people follow. The PREDIMED study of 2016 was a famous study that compared the Mediterranean diet followers' weight loss to other diet followers. The results showed that the people on the Mediterranean diet lost more weight and lost more inches in their waist circumference compared to low-fat diet followers.

The idea is to mimic the lifestyle of the people of the Mediterranean which includes their healthy diet and their active lifestyle. It's not enough if you simply follow the recipes, you also have to incorporate some activity in your life in order to see the results of weight loss. That doesn't mean you need to live at the gym, but it means making a voluntary choice to incorporate more physical activity in your day to burn calories. Physical activity can come in many forms and doesn't have to a torturous session at the gym! You can go on long walks, jog, bike, swim, or take part in cardio sessions that keep your heart rate up. This keeps your heart healthy and helps you lose and keep the weight off.

How can you take steps to begin your weight loss journey on the Mediterranean diet? Here are some suggestions.

Remember your reason for starting the Mediterranean lifestyle. Whatever your reason for starting the Mediterranean diet is, keep that in the forefront of your mind as the encouragement and motivation you need. Are you hoping to reduce your cholesterol by your next checkup? Maybe you want to lower your blood sugar levels because you have a family history of diabetes, or you want to lose some excess weight you haven't been able to get rid. Or you could have a family history of heart disease and you want to decrease the amount of red meat you consume. Whatever your reason, use that as motivation as you embrace the Mediterranean lifestyle. Whether you're looking for immediate results like weight loss or looking into the future quality of your health, your goals are important. Whatever it is, be sure you keep your goal in mind as your "why" for staying committed.

Don't stray to other diets that might seem popular at the time. When you're following one path, others may seem tempting, especially if they become popular around you. Whether it's a new juice cleanse or another diet making the rounds, you want to remind yourself why you've chosen the Mediterranean diet and why it's the one for you. Whether it's the convenience of it or the health benefits that the research has found, stay constant and don't try to find a "quick fix". With the Mediterranean diet, you're in it for the long road! It's not just a diet or exercise fad, it's a complete lifestyle mimicking the people of the Mediterranean if you hope to achieve their good health.

Start slowly by adjusting your diet if you need to. As you're doing your research on the Mediterranean diet, you will know which items you should be cutting out of your diet. And sometimes that can be tough! Whether it's processed snacks, sugar, or red meat, we are all used to certain things which may be unhealthy for us. In order to get used to the Mediterranean diet, allow yourself to gently cut back on these items if that's the approach that works for you. Going "cold turkey" can be tough, especially if you aren't an avid fish lover or have eaten processed snacks for years. Begin by cleaning out your kitchen by getting rid of what you can't eat and filling your fridge with what you can such as fresh fruits and vegetables. As long as you're able to make progress, that's a great start!

Don't overeat and consume too many calories. One of the tricky parts of the Mediterranean diet is that it doesn't give you a daily calorie count to follow. Even if you don't want to count calories, if you want to lose weight, you have to stay calorie deficit. You should be burning more calories than you consume. Your required calorie amount depends on many factors, such as gender, genetics, fitness level, body type, and health conditions. To burn calories, you have to incorporate physical activity into your routine. You can still lose weight by following the diet alone, but weight loss will be at a much slower rate. Simply by staying aware of your calories to ensure you aren't overeating you won't be at risk of putting on extra pounds.

- Eat foods with fiber. Fiber ensures that you feel full for longer, so you aren't feeling hungry for snacks between meals. Along with that, it keeps your digestive system regular. Low-calorie vegetables like cauliflower, broccoli, and Brussels sprouts are high in fiber, along with things like whole grain bread.
- Eat smaller portions. One of the things that the West has commandeered is the idea of eating huge portions of food. Pasta can take up the whole plate! But the people of the Mediterranean didn't eat that way. Their meals tended to contain portions of food such as fresh vegetables, a slice of whole grain bread, some pasta. The meal was to consist of better quality foods instead of a greater quantity. Be aware of your portion size intake and think about if you really need seconds. If you are having a diet rich in fiber, you shouldn't feel hungry soon after. Even a few extra spoonsful of food can make a difference in your daily calorie count.

- Be sure you don't eat too much fat. No matter the type of good fat the Mediterranean diet consists of, too much fat is equal to too many calories. Calories can add up, even when it's something healthy like nuts or fish. Be aware of your intake and try not to snack mindlessly because that could cause you to gain weight. Even when using olive oil, be sure you're not using an excess amount. Less is more and instead of 4 tbsp, maybe you can make do with 3 tbsp! You'll be surprised how many calories just one spoonful can contain!
- Have healthy protein. You want to make sure you have red meat rarely, but protein-rich foods are important to keep you full between meals. Also, it will help satisfy your craving for meat if you're having a hard time adjusting. Whether your protein source is fish, eggs, lentils, or beans, it's an important part of your diet to keep you full and still keep your calorie count low. Plan your diet to include fresh fish and seafood throughout the week, and you can find beans and lentils in the canned goods aisle for a quick addition to any lunch.
- Vegetables should be the focus of the meal. Like we mentioned about portion sizes, this is another aspect where the West often has often gotten it backward! We tend to keep veggies as a side in our meals with just a spoonful, but an authentic Mediterranean diet will keep vegetables the center of the dish. Even just a simple sautéed dish in olive oil with some seasoning is enough to make your vegetables delicious! Packed with vitamins, minerals, and fiber, yet still low in calories and carbohydrates.

Exercise! As we've been saying, exercise is very healthy and recommended for all individuals regardless of what diet you follow. Research has shown that physical activity can considerably lessen the chances of heart related sicknesses and improve the longevity of your life. With all these health benefits it creates, coupled with a healthy diet, it's only natural that you want to reap the benefits and spend your time doing something worthwhile. And with the Mediterranean diet, you will have the energy to do so! Unlike other diets where people drastically reduce their intake of carbohydrates which can create havoc on the body or have very small portion sizes in hopes of losing weight quickly, the Mediterranean diet includes a full and rich diet of protein and fat. That should give you the energy to get through any workout! In fact, some studies say it can give you a boost of endurance. Remember, you're mimicking the people of the Mediterranean who engage in physical activity regularly, whether it's walking somewhere, biking, swimming, or simply not taking the "shortcuts" and taking the extra steps to make them count for your health.

- Examples of aerobic exercises you can do which will increase your breathing and heart rate include: jump roping, jogging, running, biking, walking, hiking, aerobics classes, dancing, kickboxing.
- Anaerobic exercises include weight training, jumping, sprinting, heavy weight lifting, high-intensity interval training.

Manage your stress. Stress plays an important role in your health especially when it comes to fluctuations in your weight. In fact, when you are stressed, your body releases the stress hormone, cortisol, which can cause blood sugar spikes and make you feel false hunger. This can lead to other symptoms like weight gain, insomnia, mood swings, and migraines. You want to be aware of the stressful factors in your life and ensure they don't interfere with the motivation of following your new diet and exercise routine. If you are stressed, you could be tempted to break your healthy eating habits or avoid exercise.

How can you try and maintain the stress in your life?

- Find a creative outlet for your feelings that help you feel better or some sort of way to release your stress and

tension. Whether that's talking to a friend or therapist, journaling, painting, or arts and crafts.
- Add a relaxing routine to your routines such as breathing exercises, prayer, guided meditation, or yoga. This can help you manage the stress in your life and give you a relaxing routine before bedtime.
- Sleep is important so make sure you're getting a good night's rest. Have a nighttime routine and avoid screens or caffeine. Make sure your sleeping area is dark and kept cool because usually, you fall asleep faster when the temperature is cooler.
- Plan your time wisely! If you feel like you have free time throughout the day, you could be tempted to break your diet. Instead, plan out your day with activities, work, school, exercise and have a set time for meals.

Chapter 3: Disadvantages of the Mediterranean Diet

When it comes to a new diet, there may be downsides that you have to overcome. Whether it's getting familiar with new ingredients or having to be aware of your caloric intake, there are going to be challenges that you have to adjust to in order to see success in your new lifestyle. We've mentioned many of the benefits that come with the Mediterranean diet, but there are some common pitfalls to be aware of so you don't ruin the progress you've made.

The Mediterranean diet doesn't tell you exactly how much to eat! There's no exact calorie count or breakdown of protein, fat or carbohydrates like the keto diet has its followers count and track. For people who are used to strict diets where they are used to counting calories or tracking their portions, it can be tough to adjust to all the freedom! Some people love this because it allows them the freedom to plan their meals and eat a little less sometimes and a little more other times - while still following their diet! The only problem is if that leads to overeating which can be dangerous. That's why it's important to ensure you are aware of your portion sizes and how much you are eating. You don't have to count calories but you do have to avoid extra snacking and be sure you are balancing your meals with an exercise routine.

Not everyone should be drinking wine. Entwined in the Mediterranean diet is the principle of wine drinking. People who already love wine and drink it frequently may love the Mediterranean diet, even more, knowing it's encouraged! But it's important that you don't drink to excess. The idea is in moderation - that means a glass per day for the ladies, and a couple for men (who tend to have a higher body mass index). If you're drinking too much and ignoring these limits, then this can cause other health issues and could increase your risk of alcoholism. By abusing the habit, you're causing more health concerns. But not everyone can drink wine or should be. If you are on certain medication, if you have pancreatitis, if you have a history of alcoholism in your family then wine drinking is not encouraged. There are also people who choose to abstain from alcohol for religious reasons. These people are still encouraged to go on the Mediterranean diet because just the healthy diet itself can help improve your health without needing to drink wine.

It can be hard for meat-lovers to adjust. If you're someone who would eat red meat frequently throughout the week, even for multiple meals a day, the Mediterranean diet can be a tough adjustment. Just like with any diet, it always seems more tempting and delicious to want what you can't have! For people who ate red meat all the time, it can take some getting used to other sources of protein such as fish, legumes, and beans. If you're someone who hasn't experimented with seafood before, it can be a whole new experience! But the important thing is to embrace that experience and understand why it's necessary for following this diet. Red meat is linked to a higher risk of heart disease which is something that the Mediterranean diet is trying to fight. By substituting red meat for healthy protein, you can see beneficial health results like the lowering of your cholesterol, lower blood pressure, and an increase in your good cholesterol numbers. Keep these goals in mind when you miss having bacon for breakfast!

You have to be aware of your "good" fat intake. The Mediterranean diet encourages eating good fats that are healthy for your diet such as nuts, seeds, olive oil, and cheese. The problem is if you are overeating and consume too many of these fats which will, in turn, make you gain weight and increase your risk of heart disease. Since there's no rulebook or serving size to follow as a guide on the Mediterranean diet, you have to be aware of your own intake. If you are having a more than a handful of nuts as a snack, using olive oil in all your dishes, and adding some cheese or nuts as a garnish to your salad, that might too much! You have to be aware of your snacking limit to ensure you aren't consuming too many calories. Despite this worry, most people are aware of their eating habits and know that more than a handful of nuts can mean too many calories!

There's no serving count to follow. As we mentioned above that there is no caloric guide for the Mediterranean diet, there is also no daily serving count to follow. Many diets will tell you how much protein, carbohydrates, or fruits and vegetables you should be eating, and how low (or high!) your fat intake should be. If you look at the Mediterranean Food Pyramid, it uses terms like "consume often," or "consume sparingly." But there's nothing exact about that! Can you have it twice a week? What about 3 times a week? Is that too much or enough to fit the label of "often"? These terms are hard to figure out and can be tough for people who are used to a strict diet that tells you exactly how much of what to eat in a day. The most important thing is to be aware of your intake and try and have a varied menu. There are many sources of protein you should be incorporating throughout your week so you can't have the excuse of having red meat too often. Fruits and vegetables should be a part of your daily diet, so you should be looking for new combinations and delicious recipes to try. It's all about incorporating a varied diet so you are getting a variety of vitamins and minerals. Avoiding overeating and being aware of your food habits is also key!

Don't assume the diet is all pasta and bread! This is a common misconception in the West that the people of the Mediterranean's meals consist of cheesy and delicious pasta - which it can! But the truth is, the Mediterranean region never ate pasta in such large portion sizes as we do. They had maybe half a cup or 1 cup as a serving size and included other things in their meal like vegetables, whole grain bread, and fish. It was a part of their meal, not a whole plateful! If that's your assumption going into the Mediterranean diet, then you may be unpleasantly surprised to realize you have to eat more than that! It's all about a balanced diet consisting of a variety of protein sources, vegetables, whole grains, seafood, fruit, red wine, and occasionally meat and poultry. You have to incorporate everything to gain health benefits. That's why research on a diet is so important so you know what you're getting into!

People may forget they should incorporate exercise into their lifestyle. Often people become excited about trying a new diet plan and seeing the weight loss results that come with it, but they don't realize that you have to live an active lifestyle too. With this diet, you are hoping to gain the same health effects that the people of the Mediterranean live by, but you can't do that without following their diet and active lifestyle. The people there frequently incorporated exercise into their life, simply by doing things like walking, hiking, or swimming. If you are only following the Mediterranean diet and feeling like you aren't losing weight fast enough, then you are depriving yourself of exercise which could help you lose more! You can't just follow one part of their lifestyle and expect to gain the benefits!

Too much oil is not a good thing either! We've talked about the astounding benefits of olive oil and how it can combat cardiovascular disease, but just like the motto goes, too much of a good thing could end up harming you. It still counts as fat and should not be used in excess. That means you should be aware of your intake and how frequently you are using it throughout the day. If you're using it in a marinade, as well as frying and cooking and on top of your salad as a vinaigrette, that might be too much. Experts say anything from 4 to 5 tbsp a day is enough for your daily consumption. Just because it's considered more healthy and is a tenet of the Mediterranean diet doesn't mean you should be using too much.

Even with these few disadvantages that people note, this diet is still considered such a great and easy one to follow – and we've seen the countless health benefits it can bring about! It can not only improve the quality of your life, but also the longevity! With research like that and such a delicious and varied list of food groups, it's easy to see why this diet has captured the attention of millions who want to make their health a priority.

Chapter 4: Being Keen on a Mediterranean Diet

We've briefly talked about some of the disadvantages of the Mediterranean diet and why some people may have a bit of a tough time adjusting. But we have to talk about the factors that make the Mediterranean diet so appealing to the fans it has garnered all over the world - reasons other than the amazing health benefits we covered in Chapter 1! Along with the possible health benefits, here are some other reasons that many love the Mediterranean diet and have made it so popular worldwide.

There are no counting calories! This is one of those positives that people love about the Mediterranean diet. So many new diets restrict people on a calorie basis which can be quite frustrating and often detrimental to your health if you require a greater caloric intake for your physical and health needs. If you're required to count calories, you have to be very careful to remember every little thing you're eating as a snack, or even adding on your dishes like dressing or cheese. The Mediterranean diet offers a great amount of flexibility regarding this because it's shifting you away from unhealthy food choices to healthier ones. Of course, you should be aware of your dietary choices and avoid overeating, but you also have the freedom to decide on your portion sizes which means you can take an extra few veggies if you'd like, or you can skip having a snack if you're not feeling hungry. The idea is to eat more filling meals that will ensure you aren't feeling hungry other than at mealtimes. By cutting out the sugar, junk food, and fast food from your diet and loading up on fiber from fruits, vegetables, and whole grains, you're eating healthier without having to worry about every item's calorie count.

You can have wine! If you're someone who already enjoys a glass of wine to unwind after a long day, this is going to be an aspect you love about the Mediterranean diet. You get to have that glass of wine and feel good that it is allowed on your diet and can have heart-healthy properties. Recent research on red wine has found that it is high in antioxidants that may prevent cardiovascular heart disease. The people of the Mediterranean also enjoyed having red wine with a meal so it could tentatively be linked to their excellent cardiovascular health. But it's important to note many warnings regarding alcohol consumption. The Mediterranean diet encourages "moderate consumption," which means there are limits in place. Healthy men can drink 2 glasses a day. Healthy women may have up to 1 glass a day. Also, these possible health benefits are only associated with red wine - not other alcoholic beverages or hard liquor. If you're an avid drinker of those and hoping to substitute that for wine in your Mediterranean diet, that won't work! Before incorporating alcohol into your diet, you should speak to your doctor to ensure it does not interfere with your health, family history, if you're pregnant or breastfeeding, or any medication you may be taking. You don't have to be drinking wine to gain the benefits of the diet, but if you are a drinker, then you're going to love this diet even more!

The Mediterranean diet is full of fiber-rich foods so you will feel full for longer. Some diets will often restrict the amount of carbohydrates, fruit or vegetable that you can eat due to worries about too much glucose production from carbs, or natural sugars contained in fruit. Thankfully, the Mediterranean diet does no such thing! And that's a good thing because it allows you to have a diet full of fibrous foods. Beans, whole grains, lentils, and fresh vegetables are rich in fiber which is great for your body. Fiber keeps you feeling full for a longer period of time which means you are less likely to snack in between meals. That means fewer calories and more weight loss! Not only that, some diets can truly have a damaging effect on your digestive system causing constipation or diarrhea due to changes in your regular fiber intake. With the Mediterranean diet, having this high intake of fiber will keep your digestive tract functioning smoothly and keep your bowel movements regular. That means less chance of gastrointestinal or rectal problems. Fiber also gives you energy which is why many people will try and have whole grains for breakfast, such as whole grain cereal, whole wheat bread, or whole grain oatmeal.

This diet will improve your mental alertness. The Mediterranean diet removes all the processed and unhealthy substances from your diet such as refined grains, soda, fast food, trans fats, and junk food. That can be tough to do, but the results it brings are very beneficial for your body and mind. All these sugary treats would cause spikes in your blood sugar and cause a rush of insulin throughout the body. That brings around symptoms like mood swings, false hunger pants, irritability, fatigue, and weakness. Instead of keeping you mentally alert, those foods slow you down and distract you from working at your best potential. When following the Mediterranean diet, you are replacing the processed sugars with fresh vegetables and fruits that are full of healthy minerals like vitamin B, folic acid, potassium, vitamin D, omega 3 fatty acids, and more! This keeps the body functioning in top mental and cognitive functioning which gives you more alertness, focus, memory recall, and concentration.

You can have fruit which is great to satisfy your sweet tooth! Many diets forbid you from eating fruit because of their natural sugars and the net carbs that they could add to your daily caloric intake. This can be quite tough, especially if you're already giving up artificial and refined sugar. Sometimes, your sweet tooth just needs to be satisfied! The more you have to give up, often the more tempting it will be to reach for those same ingredients! With the Mediterranean diet, you're encouraged to make fruit a healthy dessert option. Instead of unhealthy sugary snacks, fruit should be your go-to. Whether it's juicy watermelon, a ripe banana, or sweet berries, these natural sugars are much less harmful to your body than artificial ones. Portion size is important so you don't want to go overboard, but many people are happy to have this option as a sweet treat!

It's very easy to adjust if you're eating outside of your home. One of the worries when you're dieting is feeling constrained if you're ever outside the comfort of your own home at mealtimes. Especially if your diet requires specialized ingredients without a lot of freedom in making meal choices at restaurants or at a friend's house. You may be panicking and wondering how to adjust. With the Mediterranean diet, it's very easy to do just that! Let's say you're out at dinner with friends. What can you order that would fit the requirements of the Mediterranean diet? Most places will offer a seafood option so you can have your choice of fish, lobster, shrimp, or crab! If there isn't a seafood choice, you can pick a poultry option - just be sure to avoid red meat! You can also pick a side of fresh vegetables or a small salad. When it comes to dessert, be sure to go for the most natural and organic option instead of a baked good full of refined sugar. You can ask for fresh fruit, or maybe an organic smoothie. The ease and flexibility that the Mediterranean diet allows even when you are outside of the home and away from your prepared meals is what makes it such a favorite among its followers. There's no panic about breaking your diet or making an unhealthy food choice.

There's so much delicious variety to choose from in the Mediterranean diet. This is not a diet you will get bored of easily or feel like the food choice is restricting. There is so much that you can eat and so many foods and recipes you can try. Remember, the Mediterranean region includes countries like Greece, Turkey, Spain, Italy, Morocco and many more! So there are always new recipes and ethnic foods that you can include in your menu. Maybe by experimenting, you'll find a new favorite! Not only that, there are great varieties of protein that you can incorporate in your dishes, as well as vegetables, whole grains, poultry, and the occasional meal of red meat. You're also encouraged to use spices, fresh herbs, and olive oil to add flavor to your meal which gives it another depth of flavor. With many avenues of exploration, you will not feel constrained by this diet or feel like you're running out of things to eat. Of course, there are clear items you should avoid like trans fats, sugar, and processed foods, but focusing on what you can eat will allow you to enjoy your meals so much more and be excited for the next one!

There will be no harmful side effects that often occur when you reduce your intake of carbohydrates. Many diets lately have been embracing the concept of low carbohydrate intake believing it causes blood sugar spikes and wanting to guide the body through a different fat-burning process called ketosis. The keto diet and other low carb diets drastically reduce the number of carbohydrates you're consuming a day. This can be a quick method to reduce weight, but it actually can bring a tough adjustment period for the body which includes symptoms like weakness, fatigue, diarrhea, muscle cramps, nausea, and other things that could interfere with your health and daily life. These are temporary, but they could still last a matter of weeks as your body adjusts. That's because carbohydrates tend to make up more than half of our diet. Cutting it down to something very minimal like 5% of your daily intake can be tough on your body! The Mediterranean diet embraces the concept of whole grains because they are healthier for you than refined carbohydrates. They're full of fiber and vitamin B12 and keep you feeling full. Whole grains tend to be lower on the glycemic index compared to refined grains. That means they will not cause blood sugar spikes. This allows you to have a more natural place for whole grains in your diet and still feel confident that you are gaining the health benefits they provide. Cutting something completely from your diet, especially something you will encounter all the time in your food choices, can be very tough and make them seem more tempting!

You don't have to become a gym rat! One of the things that people also love about the Mediterranean diet is that it doesn't require intense exercise that some diets will encourage. This makes it appealing to people of all health levels and physical fitness. It simply encourages you to incorporate more physical activity into your routine, whether that's a walk around the block, a swim session at the pool, or jogging or biking. You don't have to join an array of gym classes or feel like you're not doing enough to burn calories. The people of the Mediterranean very naturally fit exercise into their daily life and activities. They didn't end up dreading it or getting burned out which can often happen if you're following a diet where you have to devote too much time at the gym. Instead, try and make the choices to be more active voluntarily, such as taking the stairs instead of the elevator, or parking your car a few blocks away and enjoying the walk to work. This way, you're still burning calories which means you're keeping yourself healthy and losing weight at the same time!

What You Can and Cannot Eat

As with any diet, it's important to begin and plan your menu by knowing exactly what you can and cannot eat. That means knowing what's on your "allowed" list and what's on your "forbidden" list. The more informed you are, the less likely you will make a mistake and bring home something you shouldn't eat!

What You Should Be Eating Most Often:

- Vegetables: Vegetables are highly encouraged on the Mediterranean diet for the vitamins and minerals they carry, as well as fiber to keep you feeling full. Try and buy fresh vegetables, but frozen is also a good substitute. Be careful about buying canned veggies because they often are high in sodium. Be sure it's a low sodium version so you are not consuming extra salt. Ginger and garlic are considered staples in the Mediterranean diet because of the way they enhance the flavor of food and also have anti-inflammatory health benefits.

Examples) tomatoes, potatoes, green beans, bell peppers, broccoli, carrots, mushrooms, olives, squash, zucchini, spinach, kale, onions

- Fish and Seafood: This should be your main source of protein on the Mediterranean diet. You should try and include this in your diet at least two times a week - but definitely more! It is a great source of protein that will not increase your risk of heart disease, along with a high intake of omega 3 fatty acids which have been discovered to be essential for our health. There are many types of fish you can try including fatty fishes like tuna and white fish like salmon and mackerel. Try and cook them as naturally as you can and avoid fatty batters or deep frying. Simple herbs and spices should enhance the flavor.

Examples) tuna, salmon, mackerel, sardines, anchovies, clams, oysters, shrimp, lobster, mussels, crab

- Legumes and Beans: These are another great source of protein that is often overlooked. But they are full of fiber too! Not only that, they are much healthier than meat! If you're not familiar with cooking the raw version of these ingredients, then buy canned versions as long as you try and buy low sodium versions. They are great as a side or even as an addition to a healthy salad or taco.

Examples) lentils, chickpeas, beans (pinto, kidney, black, white), hummus

- Nuts and Seeds: Another category that is often overlooked, these are perfect snacks packed with healthy fats and protein. They contain omega 3 fatty acids as well as unsaturated fatty acids which are better for heart health. They are high in calories which is why you want to be aware of your intake and be sure you're not snacking mindlessly. Also, it's better if you choose unsalted or non-candy versions to ensure you're getting all the health benefits and none of the extra junk!

Examples) almonds, sunflower seeds, walnuts, hazelnuts, cashews, pumpkin seeds, pine nuts, chia seeds

- Whole Grains: These healthy carbohydrates are allowed on the Mediterranean diet because of the essential vitamins, minerals, and fiber that they add to your diet. Fiber allows you to feel full for longer and keep your digestive system regular. Whole grains are much healthier than refined grains which means your blood sugar levels will stay stable. Incorporating just a side of this in your meals or as a component of your breakfast can help keep you energized.

Examples) couscous, whole grain pasta, quinoa, rice, pita bread, Ezekiel bread, oatmeal, barley

- Extra Virgin Olive Oil: We talked about how extra virgin olive oil is such an important tenet of the Mediterranean diet. It may be a little more expensive to pay for the "extra virgin" label but just means it's the best quality of olive oil that is devoid of chemicals but still contains anti-inflammatory properties. If your olive oil has a label that says "low fat," that means it's been treated with heat to change its properties. Be sure your bottle is opaque and made of dark glass or metal because exposure to light can ruin the oil. Keep it in a dark, cool place.

Examples) avocado oil, grapeseed oil, ghee, coconut oil are allowed as acceptable alternatives, but you should try and use extra virgin olive oil for all your needs

- Fruit: The Mediterranean diet also encourages the moderate consumption of fresh fruit! Many diets prohibit it because of its natural sugar content or net carbs intake, but this diet urges you to use fruit as a natural dessert since you're forgoing refined sugar. The natural sugars found in fruit are much healthier for your body than anything artificially produced! You don't want to go overboard and eat too much a day, but make fresh fruit an option as a way to satisfy your sweet tooth or in a healthy smoothie.

Examples) bananas, apples, strawberries, melons, blueberries, dates, peaches, pears, oranges, and more!

- Herbs and Spices: This is another tenet of Mediterranean cooking which allows you to season your food and add delicious flavor without simply relying on salt or fat in your food. If you don't have access to fresh herbs in a garden or can't seem to keep them fresh for long in your fridge, dried herbs are a great alternative. Be sure to browse your herb aisle at the grocery store to try new tastes and experiment with flavors that can add a lot of depth to your dishes. The calories are negligible but the flavor is delicious!

Examples) cilantro, mint, bay leaves, basil, oregano, parsley, allspice, cloves, coriander, paprika, cumin powder, cinnamon powder, coriander powder, garam masala

What You Should Eat Moderately:
- Poultry: This is lean meat which is less harmful to your health than red meat. Fish and seafood should still make up the majority of your dishes throughout the week, but poultry is great to include as a change of pace. It's important you are aware of your portion sizes though, and use them to create low-fat dishes. Instead of making it the main meal, have it as a side with veggies or beans.

Examples) chicken, duck, turkey

- Dairy: Dairy products are very healthy for you but they should be consumed moderately because they often are high in protein as well. Too much protein can cause you to gain weight. These should be consumed moderately throughout the week so be aware of your intake to ensure you're not having too much. Try and find low-fat options if you can. You want to also focus on organic products instead of ones that are processed or contain artificial sugars or flavoring.

Examples) low-fat milk, yogurt, Greek yogurt, cheeses like mozzarella, feta, cheddar, and Parmesan

- Eggs: These should also be consumed moderately throughout the week because they are also high in protein. They make a great healthy snack though so you can have them for breakfast or a hard-boiled egg as a side for dinner. Just be aware of your intake to ensure you are not eating too many throughout the week. Buying organic or free-range is a great idea so you are exposed to fewer growth hormones.
- Red Meat: Though you should try and very sparingly eat red meat on the Mediterranean diet, it can still be put in this category because experts say your intake should be limited to around 6 to 10 oz once a week. That is a big reduction from eating it many times a week, but you could have it once a week as a "cheat meal". You should choose

lean cuts and try and buy organic for a healthier option. The more you are able to avoid this in your diet and find a healthier option like seafood or poultry, the healthier you will be.

What You Should Avoid:
- Refined Sugar and Sugary Beverages: As we've mentioned, you want to cut artificial sugars from your diet which fruit juices. Despite some fruit juices being advertised as organic, they often contain preservatives or artificial sugar mixed in for freshness. Instead, try making your own fruit smoothies with natural ingredients. And even snacks that are advertised as low in sugar can contain substitutes that will cause blood sugar spikes. It's best to avoid these and focus on natural fruit as a way to satisfy your sweet tooth.

Examples) ice cream, sugar, baked goods, fruit juices, soda, candy, sugary snacks

- Refined Grains: Whole wheat grains are encouraged on the Mediterranean diet while refined grains are unhealthy for you. They are grains where the nutrients are removed and cause unnecessary blood sugar spikes.

Examples) white bread, refined pasta, cereals, bagels, white rice, white all purpose flour

- Trans Fats and Refined Oils: Your staple on the Mediterranean diet should be extra virgin olive oil so you should other refined oils that you would have previously cooked with. Trans fats like margarine or butter are also heavily processed and have unhealthy side effects.

Examples) vegetable oil, soybean oil, canola oil, butter, shortening

- Processed Meats and Foods: These foods should be avoided on the Mediterranean diet because they have been changed so much from their original form. Even snack foods that are advertised as "low fat" or "diet friendly" tend to be highly processed with trans fats. Instead, focus on a more natural diet where you are having healthy snacks nuts, seeds, or veggies and fruit.

Examples) processed snacks, hot dogs, sausage, bacon

What You Should Drink:
- Water: This should be what you drink the most of when you're on the Mediterranean diet. It's most healthy to regulate your body and exactly what your body's tissues and cells need. You want to stay hydrated all throughout the day, not just at mealtimes, so be sure you have a water bottle with you at all times. Previously doctors would recommend 8 glasses of water a day, but recent health studies say that should be more like 12 glasses for healthy adults. If you live in an arid or dry climate, or are more physically active, it's important you have even more water. Sometimes medication can make you more thirsty as well.

- Wine: Wine is moderately allowed on the Mediterranean diet but it should be considered optional since not all people can partake in drinking alcohol. Those who take medication, have a history of alcoholism, or choose to abstain for religious reasons may have a problem with this. You should practice moderation which means no more than a glass per day for women, and 2 for men. You should talk to your doctor before including alcohol in your diet.

- Tea and Coffee: These are also allowed on the Mediterranean diet but you should be careful not to include sugar or artificial sweetener. These are empty calories and can cause your blood sugar to rise.

Even with the clear categories of what you should not be eating, it's easy to see that the Mediterranean still allows for so much diversity in your meals and snacks! That's part of what makes it appealing to its followers. With the wide range of cuisines from the Mediterranean region, many sources of protein and vegetables, there are many options for what you can make for meals. Healthy snacks are even allowed. By focusing clearly on what you can eat, you can enjoy making and experimenting with delicious recipes for a long time to come.

7 Rules for Rapid Weight Loss

A 2008 study found that participants lost more weight by following the Mediterranean diet compared to other participants who were on a low-fat diet. It's important to note that the Mediterranean diet consists of more than just olive oil, pasta, and wine. If you want to lose weight, you have to implement a balanced diet full of variety, as well as making exercise a part of your routine.

Here are some tips to help you lose weight!

Plan your meal times so you are less susceptible to snacking. No matter what diet you follow, it's important that you create a schedule and set your mealtimes. This will reduce your risk of falling hungry between meals and eating unhealthy foods in a bind. In fact, if you eat when you are extremely hungry, studies show that you end up overeating and consuming more calories than you need! Set your mealtimes based on your schedule and appetite, and allow yourself a healthy snack every 4 to 5 hours. A study in Spain found that if you tend to have lunch around 1 to 3 PM, you could reduce your risk of overeating. If you know you'll be out of the home, be sure you have healthy snacks with you so you don't give in to the temptation of fast food or a sugary snack. Veggie sticks, a whole grain sandwich, or raw nuts are great to keep nearby.

Vegetables should be your main course. Vegetables contain a moderate amount of calories and are low in carbohydrates while still keep you full of fiber, vitamins, and minerals. You want to have vegetables be the main course of your meal and it doesn't take much to make it so. You can season your food in a little olive oil, add some herbs or spices, and that's all you need! The fiber you get will keep you full for longer between meals and keep your digestive system regular. You can have some protein, whole grain bread, or fruit as a part of your meal too, but incorporate more vegetables to gain the health effects of the Mediterranean diet.

Stay hydrated. Your main source of hydration should be water which is most necessary for your body. Fruit juices contain unnecessary sugar, and you don't need as much milk because your main source of dairy will come from cheese or yogurt you consume with your dishes. Coffee and tea are allowed, but you want to ensure you are avoiding sugar or artificial sweeteners which will cause your blood sugar levels to rise. A glass of wine is allowed with a Mediterranean meal, but there is still no substitute for water and all the benefits it provides your body. To encourage yourself and keep track of your water intake, have a water bottle with you at all times and fill it up throughout the day. You can even infuse your water with fruit or mint to give it a little more flavor.

Watch your olive oil intake. Though we've talked about the many health benefits associated with olive oil, too much oil is still not good for you. It provides unnecessary calories and can increase your cholesterol, which is exactly what we don't want. Since olive oil is going to be what you use for the majority of your cooking needs, you want to ensure you aren't using too much. You shouldn't need more than 4 or 5 tbsp a day. The less you use, the better for your health!

Have more filling meals so you can avoid snacking. As we mentioned above, you want to ensure your meals are full of variety and healthy fibrous content. That means including a source of protein, like fish or beans, as well as vegetables and maybe a whole grain bread. The more fill you are after you eat, the less tempted you will be to reach for a snack in between mealtimes. You can still eat healthy snacks such as more vegetables or raw nuts, but ultimately, the fewer calories you consume, the more weight you will lose.

Stay away from the red meat and try other protein sources. The Mediterranean diet wants you to eat red meat sparingly, so the less often you include it in your meal plan, the better it will be for your health! If you are still having it regularly, then try scaling back and experimenting with more fish and seafood, as well as legumes and beans. These are low-calorie options that give you the protein you need, as well as fiber and omega 3 fatty acids. The more lean protein you eat, the more weight you will likely lose.

Get exercising! Including physical activity in your routine is important if you truly want to follow a Mediterranean lifestyle. It's not enough if you simply follow the diet and then wonder why you're not losing as much weight as you'd hoped to. If you prefer taking classes at your gym a few times a week, that is great. If you prefer to exercise in a more natural concept, then take those steps in your day such as walking places, doing housework, stretching, or gardening. These changes in your routine allow you to burn excess calories which will help you lose weight.

Chapter 5: Mindset for Success on the Mediterranean Diet

12 Tips for Success

If you're motivated at this point to begin the Mediterranean diet and see the results for yourself, we are here to give you tips for success! The more informed you are about what to expect and what changes to make, the more success you will see as you adjust your life to this new diet.

Let's get started!

1. Start using the right fats. For the Mediterranean diet, you need to make the switch to a choice of healthy oil like extra virgin olive oil. This oil is high in anti-inflammatory properties which help the body. This means making the switch in your diet and removing the unhealthy oils such as canola oil, vegetable oil, margarine or butter. Olive oil should be your go-to for all your cooking needs. Avocado oil is a good substitute as well to keep on hand. Remind yourself that "less is more," and focus on minimizing your quantity of the oil but focusing on its healthy qualities.

2. Get rid of what you can't eat. Like any diet, there will be a clear list of what you cannot eat - and the Mediterranean diet is no different. You want to get rid of those items to ensure you are not tempted. That means getting rid of the unhealthy oils, processed foods and meats, sugary snacks and juices, fast food, and junk food. Get used to having fresh ingredients on hand and allowing yourself to meal plan and prep so you have a delicious meal waiting for you. If you had a favorite dish you enjoyed, like lamb chops or fried chicken, see if you can find a Mediterranean diet alternative which is healthier for you.

3. Get used to seafood. Your main source of protein on the Mediterranean diet will be fish and seafood. If you're already a seafood lover, this is a great time to incorporate it more into your week where you would have eaten red meat. Remember, seafood is more than just fish - there's clams, shrimp, crab, lobsters, and so many other choices! It's a great addition in so many recipes whether it's served with rice, in tortillas, on top of a salad, or grilled. Not to mention the dozens of varieties of fish you can try from your local grocery store or specialized fish market store. The more variety you incorporate into your diet, the more you will be able to explore new recipes and find favorites.

4. Try other sources of protein instead of red meat. If you often had red meat throughout the week, it can be tough adjusting to other sources of protein. But it's a necessary switch and one you have to stick to, especially if you're hoping to fight symptoms of cardiovascular heart disease. Ease back on the red meat you include in your diet so you have it only sparingly. Get used to fish, seafood, chicken, beans, and legumes as a source of protein. These are low in carbs and much healthier for you. Keep meat as your "cheat meal," if you wish!

5. Make vegetables the star of your meals. You want to have a variety of vegetables on hand to incorporate it into your meals, or even as the main dish! Whether it's a healthy salad full of many vegetables, or a sautéed side of veggies with fish, it's important you are including veggies in your meals as often as you can. Fiber, vitamins and minerals which keeps us full in between meals are primarily sourced through vegetables. It also ensures that your blood sugar levels stay stable. The Mediterranean diet is all about choosing plant-based ingredients so you should try and experiment with more veggies and different ways to eat them.

6. Use herbs and spices to season your food. High sodium intake can cause health concerns and increase the risk of heart disease. Most of us are consuming too much salt and don't even realize it! Since the Mediterranean

diet is all about heart health, try and experiment with a variety of spices or herbs to add flavor your meals rather than salt. It's great to experiment with different ethnic spices and see how what kind of flavor it packs in your protein. The Mediterranean diet encompasses a whole region of countries that are along the Mediterranean sea, from Greece, Italy, Spain, to Tunisia and Morocco. There should be no shortage of recipes that you can try! Fresh herbs are also a great garnish for your meals.

7. You can choose to have wine but remember the limits you should follow. Some people love the red wine aspect of the Mediterranean diet, but it's important to remember that moderation is the key. For women, that means no more than 1 glass. 2 glasses is the maximum for men. Remember, this is only for red wine and you cannot substitute other varieties of alcohol or hard liquor. If you're not a drinker, research suggests you could even potentially get the same health benefits by snacking on grapes! Some of the same heart-healthy properties of red wine are found in grapes. So, drinking is not necessary if you are someone who has health concerns or abstains for religious reasons.

8. Make fruit your choice of dessert. We are so used to thinking of dessert as something like cake or chocolate that we don't realize the effect that has on our health. But in the Mediterranean region of the world and many others, fresh fruit is considered a dessert and is often served at the end of a meal. Whether it's ripe melons, juicy orange slices, or sweet pears, these fruits and the natural sugars they contain are much better for your health and blood sugar levels than refined or artificial sugar. Get used to having fresh fruit on hand and treating it like the dessert platter in your house. It's delicious and healthy!

9. Get moving! We've repeated over and over that the Mediterranean diet is not only a diet - it's a lifestyle change. To truly gain the benefits of the Mediterranean people, you should try and incorporate physical activity into your routine as well. If you don't like the atmosphere of a gym, that means

making voluntary choices to be more active in your day like walking, biking, swimming, hiking, performing more housework or chores around the house, etc. Whatever activity you prefer, get moving and gain the health benefits that exercise offers!

10. Plan your meals. As we mentioned before, excessive snacking can be your downfall when it comes to any diet! Even though the Mediterranean does encourage healthy snacking, the more calories you consume, the harder it will be ultimately to lose weight. It's more important to have a filling and healthy meal that will tide you over until the next mealtime! To do this, planning your meals is a great way to ensure your success. This allows you to plan, grocery shop, and prep your meals for the week. This reduces the temptation of grabbing fast food or going for something unhealthy because you know you have a meal waiting for you. Maybe use a day on the weekend to cut your veggies, marinate your fish fillets, and prepare some beans or lentils so you have them for a couple of days in advance. It helps reduce food waste, and keeps you motivated to eat what you've prepared!

11. Try and share your mealtimes with people when you can. Another wonderful thing about the Mediterranean region is their cultural tradition of eating meals together. In the West, it seems more common to have a quick "grab and go" meals alone at work or even at home. Everyone on is a different schedule and people eat when it's most convenient for them. But many believe that some of the benefits of this diet could be associated with their ritual of eating together. Research has shown that sharing a meal can improve your mood, decrease stress levels, and even control the portion size of how much you're eating! That's because you're in a social environment and everyone is slowing down to enjoy the company instead of in a hurry to quickly eat and move on. Obviously, this isn't possible with every meal every time, but it's great advice to encourage you to enjoy your food and mealtimes. So, next time, invite a colleague to eat lunch with you or invite a friend or family member over for dinner. They'll get to have a delicious meal and you'll get to enjoy their company!

12. Be flexible and embrace the possibilities! The Mediterranean diet appeals to so many because of the flexibility it gives. You don't have to count calories, count macronutrients, or drastically cut the portions of your meals. There are so many varieties of foods you can eat from fish, legumes, beans, vegetables, fruit, whole grains, poultry, dairy, and seafood. This gives you such variety in your meals so that you can experiment with new recipes and new cuisines. Don't allow yourself to get bored when there are so many options available and new combinations you can try. As long as you are staying away from the unhealthy items and sparingly consuming red meat, you can allow yourself a delicious diet full of meals you love.

Chapter 6: 14 Day Sample Meal Plan

To get you started on your Mediterranean diet, we have a 14-day sample meal plan prepared for you to show you how easy and delicious these recipes can be! There are no specialty ingredients you have to buy – just keeping a fresh stock of herbs, vegetables, pasta, and fish and seafood, with the occasional meat dish allowed. Quick and easy, these are great recipes to get you started and falling in love with this diet!

MONDAY
Breakfast: Mediterranean Frittata
3 servings total, 109 calories per serving, 9 grams protein, 7 grams fat, 3 grams carbs

Ingredients:
a pinch of salt, black pepper, and paprika
2 tbsp cheese (Feta), crumbled
8-10 olives, sliced
.25 cup tomatoes, diced
.25 cup milk or heavy cream
3 eggs

Directions:
Pre-heat your oven to 400 degrees. Lightly use a few drops of olive oil or cooking spray to grease a pie or quiche dish. Combine your eggs and milk and incorporate the other ingredients. Bake until the eggs are set for about 15 to 20 minutes.

Lunch: Chickpea and Chicken Salad
3 servings total, 221 calories per serving, 22 grams carbs, 8 grams fat, 20 grams protein, 4 grams fiber

Ingredients:

8-10 olives, sliced
3-4 fresh basil leaves, chopped
1 can chickpeas (~15 oz)
2 tbsp cheese (Feta), crumbled
2 tbsp olive oil
1 cup cooked and shredded chicken breast
.5 head lettuce, chopped
1 tomato, chopped
1 tspn lemon or lime juice

Directions:
Mix the olive oil, lemon juice, and basil to make your salad dressing. Combine the rest of your vegetable ingredients and mix with the dressing. Season with a little salt and pepper if preferred

Dinner: Sautéed Shrimp and Asparagus
4 servings total, 302 calories per serving, 6 grams fat, 34 grams carbs, 28 grams protein

Ingredients:
8-10 spears of fresh asparagus
.25 cup green onions, chopped
2 tspn olive oil
1 pound fresh or frozen peeled shrimp
4 cloves garlic, minced
salt, black pepper, and paprika to taste
.25 cup dry red wine
.25 cup green onions, chopped
1" ginger root, minced

Directions:
Add your olive oil in a pan, and saute your shrimp in it once it is hot. Season with the ginger, garlic, salt, and black pepper. Next, pour in the wine. Add

the asparagus and let it cook. Once the asparagus stems are tender, add the green onions to the skillet. You can serve with a side of rice or pasta.

TUESDAY
Breakfast: Mediterranean Scrambled Eggs
2 servings total, 248 calories per serving, 17 grams fat, 13 grams carbs, 2.8 grams fiber, 17 grams protein

Ingredients:
1 tablespoon olive oil
3-4 black olives, sliced
6 cherry tomatoes, sliced
1 yellow pepper, diced
4 eggs
.25 tspn dried oregano
2 spring onions, sliced
a dash of salt and black pepper

Directions:
On medium flame, heat the olive oil in a pan. Add your spring onions and pepper and sauté until the vegetables become soft. Then add the tomatoes and olives. Crack your eggs into the pan and scramble them so they are cooked through. Add the salt, black pepper, and oregano. Keep stirring until the eggs are cooked and remove from heat.

Lunch: Greek Yogurt Chicken Stuffed Peppers
6 servings total, 118 calories per serving, 18 grams carbs, 3 grams fat, 9 grams protein

Ingredients:
.5 cup Greek yogurt
8-10 cherry tomatoes, chopped
.5 cucumber, chopped

2 tbsp fresh parsley, chopped
3 bell peppers, halved, seeds removed
salt and black pepper to taste
chicken from 1 rotisserie chicken, shredded
.25 cup celery, chopped
1 tspn rice vinegar
1 tablespoon mustard

Directions:
In a bowl, combine the rice vinegar, mustard, and Greek yogurt, and season with salt and black pepper. Add the cucumber, celery, parsley, tomatoes, and chicken and stir until well coated in the yogurt. Divide the chicken yogurt mixture into the 6 portions of the bell pepper. Garnish with the parsley.

Dinner: Lime Salmon
2 servings total, 354 calories per serving, 16 grams fat, 34 grams protein, 12 grams carbs

Ingredients:
6 tspn olive oil, divided
3 tspn fresh parsley, chopped
2 salmon fillets
salt and black pepper to taste
2 tspn lemon juice
1 tspn dried oregano herbs

Directions:
Marinade your salmon with salt, black pepper, and half the lemon juice. In a pan on medium heat, add about 2 tspn of the olive oil. Once hot, add your salmon fillets skin side up. Cook until light and flaky. In a separate container, mix the remaining olive oil. Drizzle that over the salmon and cook for another few minutes on both sides. Garnish with fresh parsley.

WEDNESDAY
Breakfast: Mediterranean Egg Muffins with Ham
6 servings total, 110 calories per serving, 6.9 grams fat, 1.8 grams carbs, 1.8 grams fiber, 10 grams protein

Ingredients:
.25 cup cheese (Feta), crumbled
.25 cup fresh spinach, minced
3-4 pieces of fresh basil, minced
5 eggs
a pinch of salt and black pepper
2 tbsp pesto sauce
.5 bell pepper, sliced
7-8 slices deli ham

Directions:
Pre-heat your oven to 400 degrees F. Use a few drops of olive oil or olive oil spray to grease your muffin tins. Place some ham at the bottom of each tin, then add the bell pepper, spinach and feta cheese on top. In a bowl, mix your eggs and season. You can pour your mixture between your 6 muffin tins and bake for 1about 15 minutes until the eggs are set. Garnish with some pesto sauce and basil

Lunch: Mediterranean Baked Zucchini Sticks
4 servings total, 1 stick zucchini per serving, 30 calories per serving, 2 grams fat, 3 grams carbs, 1.8 grams protein

Ingredients:
2 medium zucchinis, sliced lengthwise down the middle
.25 cup olives, chopped
.25 cup tomatoes, chopped
1 tspn dried oregano
.25 cup parsley, chopped

salt and black pepper to taste
2 oz cheese (Feta), crumbled
.25 cup bell pepper, chopped
1 tspn minced garlic

Directions:
Set your oven to 350 degrees F. Use a large spoon to remove the flesh of the zucchini. You can eat or discard the flesh. Combine the vegetables you have prepared and season with black pepper, oregano, and salt. Spoon some of the mixture into each of the 4 zucchini "boats". On a baking tray, arrange the zucchini boats and bake for about 15 minutes. Then sprinkle on the feta cheese and you can broil for an additional couple of minutes. Garnish with fresh parsley.

Dinner: Greek Lamb Chops
4 servings total, 197 calories per serving, 9 grams fat, 25.2 grams protein, 3 grams carbs

Ingredients:
3 tspn olive oil
2 tspn dried oregano
8 lamb loin chops, fat trimmed
2 tspn lemon juice
2 tspn minced garlic
salt and black pepper to taste

1 tablespoon red wine vinegar
1 tspn dried basil

Directions:
Combine the dried herbs, vinegar, garlic, and lemon juice and season with salt and black pepper. You want to rub your lamb chops with this marinade. Rub a baking tray with the olive oil so it is coated and then add the lamb

chops. Broil on low flame for around 10 minutes on each side until cooked to your level of done.

THURSDAY
Breakfast: Feta Frozen Yogurt
3 servings total, 168 calories per serving, 10 grams fat, 12 grams carbs, 6.7 grams protein

Ingredients:
.5 cup cheese (Feta)
1 cup Greek yogurt
Honey (optional)

Directions:
Combine all the ingredients in a blender or food processor and pour into a dish. Freeze until solid the night before. Garnish with fresh nuts to eat the next morning.

Lunch: Lentil Greek Salad
4 servings total, 104 calories per serving, 3 grams fat, 20 grams carbs, 7 grams protein

Ingredients:
.75 cup dry brown lentils
1 bay leaf
1 tspn garlic, minced
.25 cup red onion, finely diced
.25 cup bell pepper, finely diced
3 tbsp fresh parsley, minced
.5 cup carrots, finely diced
.5 cup celery, chopped
3 tbsp lemon juice
pinch of salt and black pepper
1 tablespoon olive oil

Directions:
In a saucepan, add the bay leaf and lentils. Add water so that the lentils are completely covered. You want to cook the lentils until they are soft by raising the heat then letting it simmer. This can take about 13 to 16 minutes. You want them soft but not mushy. Drain the water and throw away the bay leaf. Add the lentils to a bowl and combine with the other chopped veggies, garlic, olive oil, and lemon juice. Season with salt and black pepper. Stir until everything well combined.

Dinner: Grilled Fish and Avocado Tacos
2 servings total, 376 calories per serving, 18 grams fat, 30 grams carbs, 27 grams protein

Ingredients:
4 whole wheat tortillas
2 tbsp fresh parsley, chopped
4 tbsp Greek yogurt
.5 avocado
1 pound codfish (or tilapia or mahi-mahi)
3 tbsp olive oil, divided
1 tspn ground cumin powder
1 tspn chili powder
.5 tspn minced garlic
3 tbsp lemon juice, divided

Directions:
Combine about half of the lemon juice and olive oil mixtures with the chili powder, cumin powder, and minced garlic in a bowl. Rub into the codfish until it's well coated. Pre-heat your grill or grill pan and grill your fish until cooked. Add the rest of the olive oil and lemon juice in a bowl, whisk thoroughly. Drizzle that to the avocado, place that on the grill. Once cooked, cut into slices. Add the shredded fish, yogurt, avocado slices into the tortillas.

FRIDAY
Breakfast: Green Smoothie with Avocado and Apple
2 servings total, 422 calories per serving, 21 grams fat, 55 grams carbs, 9 grams protein

Ingredients:
1 banana, frozen for 15 minutes
3 tbsp chia seeds
1 avocado
2 cups of coconut water
1 Granny Smith apple, chopped
3 cups spinach

Directions:
In a blender, mix the coconut water, spinach, and apple and blend, check if the consistency is smooth. Then add in the other ingredients and continue to blend until everything is of the same consistency.

Lunch: Chicken Salad Panini Sandwiches
2 servings total, 1 sandwich per serving, 285 calories per serving, 12 grams fat, 20 grams carbs, 24 grams protein

Ingredients:
2 slices provolone cheese
1 tspn olive oil
.25 cup roasted red peppers, drained and cut
2 tspn mayonnaise
.25 cup spinach or arugula leaves
4 slices whole wheat bread
2 tspn garlic, minced
.5 cup cooked chicken breast, chopped
1 tablespoon red wine vinegar

Directions:
Mix together the minced garlic, mayonnaise, vinegar, and chicken. Spoon out the chicken mixture on the 4 slices of bread and top with your arugula or spinach leaves, pepper, and cheese. Apply the olive oil to a panini grill or indoor grill and follow the instructions to cook the sandwiches until toasted.

Dinner: Spicy Crab Pasta
4 servings total, 362 calories per serving, 13 grams fat, 46 grams carbs, 13 grams protein

Ingredients:
.5 package bow tie (farfalle) pasta ~16 oz
salt and black pepper to taste
1 tspn red chili flakes
3 tspn olive oil
2 tspn minced garlic
2 tomatoes, diced
1 can crab meat, drained ~6 ounce

Directions:
Using bigger pot, prepare your pasta based on the directions given in the packaging. The consistency of the paste would also be dependent in your personal taste or preference. In another pot, add your olive oil first. Then the crab meat and tomatoes. Add your seasonings of chili flakes, black pepper, and salt. Mix with the pasta to serve.

SATURDAY
Breakfast: Mediterranean Toast

1 serving total, 321 calories per serving, 33 grams carbs, 16 grams protein, 8 grams fiber, 17 grams fat

Ingredients:
.25 avocado, mashed
1 tablespoon hummus
1 hardboiled egg
2 tspn cheese (Feta), crumbled
1 slice whole wheat bread
salt and black pepper to taste
3 cherry tomatoes, sliced

Directions:
First, toast your slice of bread if you prefer and slice your hard-boiled egg. Spread the hummus and avocado and arrange your tomato slices, hardboiled egg, and top with feta cheese. Season with salt and black pepper.

Lunch: Greek Style Chicken Salad
4 servings total, 220 calories per serving, 9 grams fat, 24 grams protein, 15 grams carbs

Ingredients:
2 cups shredded chicken
2 tomatoes, diced
1 large cucumber, diced
5 cups romaine lettuce, torn into pieces
zest and juice of 1 lemon
.5 cup Greek vinaigrette salad dressing
.5 cup onion, chopped
.25 cup olives, halved
.5 cup bell pepper, chopped
.5 cup cheese (Feta), crumbled
.5 tspn dried oregano

Directions:
To make your dressing, combine half of the vinaigrette, oregano, and the lemon zest. Then add lettuce, cucumber, tomatoes, bell pepper, onion, chicken, olives, and feta cheese. Add the lemon juice and the dressing.

Dinner: Greek Lemon Chicken and Potatoes
4 servings total, 1138 calories per serving, 75 grams fat, 35 grams carbs, 80 grams protein

Ingredients:
4 chicken thighs
1 tspn dried rosemary
.5 cup fresh lemon juice
.25 cup olive oil
2 tspn garlic, minced
1 tspn salt
1 tspn paprika
3 russet potatoes, peeled and diced
1 tspn black pepper
.5 cup chicken broth

Directions:
Set your oven to 425 degrees F. Lightly spread olive oil on the roasting pan to grease it. Combine the salt, black pepper, paprika, garlic, rosemary, lemon juice, and olive oil as a marinade for the chicken. Rub over the chicken pieces, and add the potato until everything is evenly coated. On a prepared roasting pan, place your chicken skin side up, and then scatter potato pieces among them. Drizzle with the chicken broth and add the rest of the marinade. Bake for 15 to 20 minutes, then give the pan a toss and cook for another 15 minutes. You can take out your chicken and then broil your potatoes lightly if you prefer a golden color.

SUNDAY
Breakfast: Chia and Berry Overnight Oats
1 serving total, 560 calories per serving, 22 grams fat, 76 grams carbs, 20 grams protein

Ingredients:
.5 cup rolled oats
1 cup of frozen berries
pinch of salt and cinnamon
1 cup milk
.25 cup chia seeds

Directions:
In a container with a lid or a Mason jar, combine your oats, milk, salt, cinnamon, and chia seeds. Puree the berries and add to the top of the oats. You can add yogurt or more berries.

Lunch: Chicken and Mozzarella Melts
4 servings total, 1 sandwich per serving, 300 calories per serving, 10 grams fat, 20 grams carbohydrates, 32 grams protein

Ingredients:
2 sweet peppers, sliced
4 skinless chicken thighs
1 cup spaghetti sauce
4 slices whole grain Italian bread
3-4 fresh basil leaves, sliced
.5 cup mozzarella cheese
8-10 olives, sliced
.5 tspn dried rosemary or oregano
3 tbsp grated Parmesan cheese

Directions:
First, cook your chicken (either a slow cooker, on the stove, or on a skillet) again it depends on what is available to you and according to your preference. Cook with the spaghetti sauce, rosemary, and sweet peppers so the chicken becomes soft and can be shredded. Then lay out your slices of bread on a baking tray. Transfer the chicken mixture onto the bread. Top with olives, basil, and Parmesan and mozzarella cheese (save some cheese!). Broil in the oven for a few minutes so your cheese becomes lightly golden. Flip over and add the chicken mixture to the other side. Sprinkle with leftover cheese and broil again for a few minutes.

Dinner: Salmon and Couscous Casserole
4 servings total, 332 calories per serving, 9 grams fat, 30 grams fat, 32 grams carbohydrates

Ingredients:
3 tspn garlic, minced
2 cups fresh baby spinach
.75 cup whole wheat couscous
1 can salmon, drained ~15 oz
.5 cup red sweet peppers from a jar, drained and chopped
3 tbsp bruschetta mixture
2 tbsp almonds
1 cup of water

Directions:
Using a microwavable dish, add the water and garlic. You can heat the water in the microwave until it is boiling, or do on the stove. Add the salmon mixture and couscous. Let it rest for about 6 to 8 minutes. Wait until the couscous is cooked. Now it's time to add your other ingredients – the bruschetta, peppers, and spinach. Mix everything until well combined and then you can top with almonds as a garnish for some crunch.

MONDAY
Breakfast: Avocado & Egg Breakfast Sandwich
1 serving total, 307 calories per serving, 11 grams protein, 7.9 grams fiber, 29 grams carbs, 16 grams fat,

Ingredients:
1 tspn olive oil
2 slices whole wheat bread
6-8 asparagus stems, steamed
.5 avocado, mashed
1 tspn mustard
1 hardboiled egg

Directions:
Toast your bread then spread the mustard and mashed avocado. Arrange your asparagus and the hard-boiled egg slices. If you prefer, you can sprinkle some salt and black pepper and a few drops of olive oil.

Lunch: Zucchini and Lemon Noodles
2 servings total, 199 calories per serving, 19.8 grams fat, 8 grams carbs, 1.9 grams protein

Ingredients:
zest of half a lemon
1 tspn olive oil
2 small zucchinis made into noodles or pre-packaged zucchini noodles
2 tspn lemon juice
.5 tspn garlic powder
3-4 radishes, sliced
1 tablespoon fresh thyme, chopped
.5 tspn mustard

Directions:
In a bowl, prepare your dressing first – combine the garlic powder, olive oil, lemon juice and the lemon zest, and the mustard. In another bowl, combine the zucchini noodles. Drizzle the olive oil dressing you just made. Garnish with the fresh thyme and radishes.

Dinner: Lentil Soup
4 servings total, 257 calories per serving, 34 grams carbs, 6 grams fat, 14 grams protein

Ingredients:
1 onion, diced
2 tspn olive oil
.75 cup lentils, soaked, rinsed
1 bay leaf
2 tspn garlic, minced
1 celery, diced
1 cup chicken stock
.5 cup carrots, diced
1 cup crushed tomatoes
.25 cup Parmesan cheese, grated
.25 cup white wine
1 tspn salt, paprika, and black pepper

Directions:
Add olive oil to a pot to sauté the onions until golden brown then you can add the following vegetables: carrots, celery, and garlic. Let those veggies soften then add the tomatoes, lentils, bay leaf, and chicken stock. Season with your spices before adding the wine and bringing the mixture to a boil. Let it simmer for 20-30 minutes. Garnish with Parmesan cheese.

TUESDAY
Breakfast: Date and Almond Smoothie
1 serving total, 421 calories per serving, 7 grams protein, 80 grams carbs, 13 grams fat

Ingredients:
1 banana
.25 cup dates, pitted
.75 cup almond milk, unsweetened
a handful of ice
1 tablespoon almond butter

Directions:
Let the dates soak in the almond milk until they are softened for about 10 to 15 minutes (or leave overnight in the fridge). Combine the ingredients and blend until it has a smooth consistency.

Lunch: Falafel Burger
1 serving total, 343 calories per serving, 6 grams fat, 61 grams carbs, 10 grams protein

Ingredients:
1 ready-made falafel patty
1 whole grain hamburger bun
1 tspn olive oil
1 lettuce leaf
1-2tspn tzatziki sauce
2-3 thin slices of red onion
2-3 tomato slices

Directions:
You can lightly pan fry your falafel in a little bit of olive oil. It should be cooked through in a few minutes. Drain any excess oil on a paper towel

before making your burger. Add the vegetables as a topping and the tzatziki sauce.

Dinner: Greek Lemon Chicken Soup
4 servings total, 221 calories per serving, 8 grams fat, 22 grams carbs, 11 grams protein

Ingredients:
1 boneless chicken breast
3 tbsp chives, chopped
2 tbsp cheese (Feta), crumbled
.5 cup couscous
1 tablespoon garlic, minced
1.5 tablespoon olive oil
.5 sweet onion, chopped
4-5 cups chicken broth
salt, black pepper, and paprika to taste
1 tablespoon lemon juice
1 tspn lemon zest for flavor

Directions:
Begin by adding olive oil to a large pot. Once your oil is hot, then sautéyour onion and garlic. Once it's fragrant and translucent, add broth and the chicken. Then it's time to add your seasonings to the meat - salt, black pepper, lemon zest, and paprika. Bring to boil then let it simmer before adding the couscous and additional salt to taste. Simmer for 5-9 minutes. Use tongs or a fork to shred the chicken.

WEDNESDAY
Breakfast: Mediterranean Omelet
1 serving total, 300 calories per serving, 20 grams carbs, 18 grams fat, 17 grams protein

Ingredients:
1 tablespoon feta cheese
2 eggs
1 artichoke, chopped
1 small tomato, chopped
4-5 olives, sliced
1 tablespoon milk
2 tspn pesto sauce
1 tspn olive oil
a dash of fresh herbs for flavor
salt and black pepper to taste

Directions: Crack your eggs into a bowl and season with salt and black pepper. Add the olive oil to a pan on medium heat then add the egg mixture and spread it out. Once the eggs set, add your cheese and vegetables and fold the egg. Garnish with pesto sauce once removing from heat.

Lunch: White Bean Salad with Tomato & Cucumber
2 servings total, 2 cups per serving, 253 calories per serving, 15 grams fat, 22 grams carbs, 8 grams protein

Ingredients:
pinch of salt and black pepper
10-12 basil leaves, chopped
3 cups mixed salad greens
1 can low sodium cannellini beans ~15 oz
1 cup cherry tomatoes, halved
1 tspn mustard
1 tablespoon red wine vinegar
2 tbsp olive oil
.5 cucumber, diced
2 tbsp onion, chopped
Directions:

Using a food processor or blender – combine your basil, vinegar, olive oil, mustard, salt, black pepper process until it has a smooth consistency. This will be your dressing. In a large bowl, you will want to combine your salad ingredients – the greens, tomatoes, cucumber, onion, and beans. Add the dressing and mix well.

Dinner: Lemon Pepper Salmon
2 servings total, 239 calories per serving, 17 grams fat, 20 grams protein, 1 gram carbs

Ingredients:
salt and black pepper to taste
2 salmon fillets ~4 oz each
3 tspn olive oil
2 tbsp low sodium soy sauce
2 tspn red wine vinegar
1 tspn tomato sauce
1 tablespoon lemon juice

Directions:
Grease a baking sheet with a few drops of olive oil. Set the salmon fillets on the baking tray. Combine the liquids as a marinade and season with salt and black pepper, then brush over the salmon. Broil for 6 to 9 minutes.

THURSDAY
Breakfast: Egg White Scramble with Veggies
2 servings total, 149 calories per serving, 16 grams protein, 7 grams carbs, 6 grams fat

Ingredients:
3 tbsp parmesan cheese, shredded
.25 cup cherry tomatoes, halved
2 tspn red onion, finely diced

1 cup fresh baby spinach
salt and black pepper to taste
.25 cup milk
6 egg whites or 1.5 cups refrigerated egg product
2 cloves garlic, minced
3 tbsp olive oil

Directions:
In a bowl, combine your milk and eggs and season the mixture. In a large frying pan, add olive oil then add the garlic. Add the vegetables and cook until the spinach becomes wilted. Then remove from heat and add your egg mixture. Cook your eggs then remove from heat and serve with veggies. Top with the shredded cheese.

Lunch: Pita Bread, Hummus, and Greek Salad
1 serving total, 414 calories per serving, 30 grams fat, 28 grams carbs, 10 grams protein, 6 grams fiber

Ingredients:
.25 cup hummus
1 whole wheat pita bread
1 tbsp cheese (Feta), crumbled
1.5 cups arugula
.5 cucumber, diced
.5 cup carrot, chopped
1 tablespoon red wine vinegar
3 tspn olive oil
1 tomato, diced
pinch of salt and black pepper

Directions:
In a large salad bowl, mix the cucumber, carrots, oil, red wine vinegar, arugula, tomatoes, and feta cheese. Eat with a side of pita bread and hummus.

Dinner: Parmesan and Lemon Chicken with Zucchini Noodles
2 servings total, 632 calories per serving, 36 grams fat, 4 grams carbs, 70 grams protein

Ingredients:
1 package of zucchini noodles
salt and black pepper to taste
.25 cup parmesan cheese, grated
2 boneless chicken breasts, cubed
2 tspn minced garlic
2 tbsp olive oil
1 tspn dried oregano
.5 cup chicken or veggie broth
2 tspn lemon zest
.5 tspn dried basil

Directions:
Cook and drain the zucchini noodles according to the instructions. Add the olive oil and cook the chicken in a separate pan. Season with salt and black pepper. Remove the chicken once cooked but keep the heat on and add the garlic, lemon zest, basil, oregano, and your broth of choice. Let the mixture cook well before you let it cook on low to medium heat. Add the chicken back to the pan and let the dish cook until the sauce has reduced. Serve with the zucchini noodles.

FRIDAY
Breakfast: Herb and Egg Frittata

1 serving total, 265 calories per serving, 18 grams carbs, 22 grams protein, 12 grams fat

Ingredients:
2 egg whites
.5 cup onion, diced
1 tspn olive oil
.25 cup water
salt and black pepper to taste
3 tspn ricotta cheese
1 tspn dried herbs (or 2 tspn if you are using fresh ones)

Directions:
Add water to a saucepan first and let it come to a boil. Add the olive oil and cook the onions first. Then crack in the eggs and cook with salt, pepper, and herbs seasoning. Garnish with cheese and remove from heat.

Lunch: Mediterranean Salad Bowl

2 servings total, 108 calories per serving, 7 grams fat, 7 grams carbs, 5 grams protein

Ingredients:
.25 cup zucchini, chopped
.5 cup bell pepper, chopped
.5 cup broccoli
2 tbsp cheese (Feta), crumbled
2 tbsp red wine vinegar
1 cup romaine lettuce, torn
1 tomato, chopped
.5 cucumber, chopped
1 tablespoon pesto

Directions:
Mix your pesto and red wine vinegar to make your salad dressing. In a salad bowl, combine all your other veggies and garnish with the feta cheese. Add the vinaigrette.

Dinner: Garlic Shrimp
4 servings total, 248 calories per serving, 14 grams fat, 17 grams protein, 7.3 grams carbs

Ingredients:
1 pound large shrimp, peeled
.25 cup olive oil
2.5 tspn minced garlic
.5 tspn chili flakes
.5 tspn paprika
1 tspn salt
2 tbsp red wine vinegar
2 tbsp lemon juice
1 tablespoon fresh parsley, chopped

Directions:
n a large pan, add the olive oil then add the garlic and chili flakes once it is hot. Be sure the garlic doesn't burn! Add in your shrimp and then season with paprika and salt. Cook for up to 5 minutes until they are no longer raw and turn pink in color. Add your liquids of lemon juice and vinegar and let them cook and reduce. Remove from heat and garnish with parsley.

SATURDAY
Breakfast: Multi Grain Breakfast Sandwich
1 serving total, 239 calories per serving, 12 grams fat, 27 grams carbs, 13.4 grams protein

Ingredients:
1 tspn olive oil
4-5 fresh baby spinach leaves
pinch of salt and black pepper
1 multi-grain sandwich bagel
2 eggs
2-3 cherry tomatoes, sliced

Directions:
Pre-heat your oven to 375 degrees F. Spread a little olive oil on the sandwich thins and toast them in the oven until lightly golden brown. In a skillet, cook the eggs in the rest of the olive oil. Once cooked, set aside. Add the tomatoes, baby spinach and egg on each bagel thin, and sprinkle with salt and black pepper.

Lunch: Shrimp Tortilla
1 serving total, 365 calories per serving, 26 grams protein, 12 grams fat

Ingredients:
4 oz cooked shrimp, roughly chopped
.5 tomato, diced
.25 avocado, diced
1 whole wheat tortilla
2 tspn lemon juice
1 tablespoon onion, chopped
.5 cucumber, chopped
2 oz cheese (Feta), crumbled

Directions:
In a bowl, mix together the tomatoes, feta, cucumber, shrimp, avocado, lemon juice, and onion. Heat your tortilla and add the filling to eat as a wrap.

Dinner: Shrimp Scampi Skewers
4 servings total, 327 calories per serving, 30 grams carbs, 36 grams protein, 7 grams fat

Ingredients:
2 tspn minced garlic
1 pound large shrimp, peeled
4 oz whole wheat vermicelli pasta
1 tspn salt
1 tspn paprika
2 tbsp of olive oil
.5 bunch of fresh parsley, chopped
1 tspn lemon juice
1 tspn black pepper

Directions:
First, season your shrimp with your spices. Thread them onto 4 skewers of about 8-10" long. Prepare your gas or coal grill and grill the skewers, being sure to turn them once so both sides are even. Cook your pasta according to the instructions. Add the shrimp skewers to the pasta dish and garnish with lemon juice and parsley.

SUNDAY
Breakfast: Oats with Fruit
1 serving total, 532 calories per serving, 19 grams fat, 75 grams carbs, 18 grams protein

Ingredients:
.25 cup fresh raspberries
.5 cup milk
.5 cup yogurt
.25 cup chopped raw nuts of your choice
.5 cup oats

a pinch of cinnamon powder

Directions:
In a jar with a lid, mix the oats, a pinch of cinnamon and the milk. Let it chill overnight or for a few hours. Then add your fruit, yogurt, and nuts as a topping before eating.

Lunch: Mediterranean Tuna Salad
3 servings total, 139 calories per serving, 8 grams fat, 11 grams carbs, 11.5 grams protein

Ingredients:
.25 cup chickpeas
7-9 black olives, sliced
.25 cup onion, finely minced
.5 cup bell pepper, chopped
.5 cucumber, diced
1 tablespoon lemon juice
1 can of tuna fish, drained ~6 oz
3 cloves garlic, minced
3 tablespoon olive oil
.5 cup carrots, diced

Directions:
In a bowl, mix together your tuna with the garlic, chickpeas, pepper, olives, carrots, onions, and cucumber. Mix in your lemon juice and olive oil to make the dressing. Add a pinch of black pepper or salt and garnish with parsley

Dinner: Kale and Feta Pasta
4 servings total, 269 calories per serving, 22 grams fat, 13 grams carbs, 7 grams protein

Ingredients:
3 cloves garlic, minced
1 package fettuccine pasta
5 tbsp olive oil, divided
4 tbsp cheese (Feta), crumbled
salt and black pepper to taste
8-10 cherry tomatoes, halved
4 cups of water
6-7 cups fresh kale leaves

Directions:
Add half the olive oil to a large pot. Then you want to stir in your kale leaves on medium heat. They will become wilted in just a few minutes so remove from the pan. Next, add the pasta, the water, tomatoes, garlic, and salt and pepper and cook on medium to high heat. Simmer until the pasta is finished cooking then season with the cheese and olive oil.

Chapter 7: Mediterranean Diet Breakfast Recipes

Banana Overnight Oats
1 serving total, 540 calories per serving, 9 grams fiber, 18 grams protein, 61 grams carbs, 21 grams fat

Ingredients:
.5 tspn cinnamon
1 tspn chia seeds
.5 cup milk
.5 cup rolled oats
2 tbsp peanut butter
.25 tspn vanilla extract
.25 cup bananas, sliced

Directions:
Add the oats, vanilla, cinnamon, and chia seeds to a container with a lid. Layer the banana and peanut butter one spoon at a time. Refrigerate for a few hours.

Mediterranean Quinoa Breakfast Bowl
3 servings total, 352 calories per serving, 20 grams fat, 20 grams carbs, 22 grams protein

Ingredients:
6 eggs
salt and black pepper to taste
.25 cup cherry tomatoes, halved
.25 cup cheese (Feta), crumbled
1 cup cooked quinoa
.25 cup yogurt
1 tspn garlic, minced
1.5 cup fresh baby spinach

1 tablespoon olive oil

Directions:
Mix together your eggs, garlic, salt, black pepper, and yogurt. Cook your spinach in the olive oil and stir until wilted Add the tomatoes. Once they are soft, add your egg mixture and cook until your eggs are done. Keep stirring so your eggs become scrambled. Add your cooked quinoa and feta cheese to the pan so they become warm too. Remove from heat.

Mediterranean Breakfast Burrito
3 servings total, 250 calories per serving, 11 grams fat, 21 grams carbs, 1.8 grams fiber, 13.9 grams protein

Ingredients:
3 whole wheat tortilla
.5 cup beans of your choice
1 tablespoon sun-dried tomatoes
.25 cup cheese (Feta), crumbled
6-8 olives, sliced
1 cup fresh baby spinach
4 eggs

Directions:
In a small frying pan, scramble your eggs until they are cooked. Add the sun-dried tomatoes, olives, and spinach. Add feta cheese and take off the heat. Add beans to each tortilla and divide the egg mixture into each one. Wrap and then grill on a frying pan or a panini press.

Healthy Breakfast Bowl
1 serving total, 421 calories per serving, 27 grams fat, 81 grams carbs, 14 grams protein

Ingredients:
.5 banana, sliced
.5 cup Greek yogurt
1 tspn chia seeds
2-3 strawberries, sliced
.5 cup raspberries
1 tablespoon almond butter
2 tbsp blueberries

Directions:
Let your chia seeds soak in your Greek yogurt overnight or for a few hours if you can. Make your raspberry compote by placing the raspberries in a small saucepan on the stove. Stir the mixture until it has liquefied then remove from heat. You can also heat in the microwave but be sure to stir in 10 to 15-second intervals. Add your sliced banana and strawberries to the yogurt and top with the almond butter and raspberry compote.

Berry Chia Overnight Oats
1 serving total, 562 calories per serving, 22 grams fat, 76 grams carbs, 20 grams protein

Ingredients:
1 cup frozen berries of your choice
extra berries for topping
.5 cup rolled oats
.25 cup chia seeds
1 cup milk
pinch of salt and cinnamon

Directions:
Combine your milk, chia seeds, oats, salt and cinnamon in Mason jars with lid or containers with a lid. Let refrigerate overnight or for a few hours. Puree the berries for a nice texture. Add extra toppings if you prefer.

Slow Cooker Mediterranean Frittata
3 servings total, 167 calories per serving, 11 grams fat, 4 grams carbs, 12 grams protein

Ingredients:
6 eggs
.25 cup milk
1 cup chopped red peppers
s.5 onion, thinly sliced
2 cups arugula
.5 cup goat cheese or feta cheese
1 tspn dried oregano
1 tablespoon olive oil
salt and pepper to taste

Directions:
Grease your slow cooker with a little bit of olive oil or use a slow cooker liner if you use those. Combine your milk, eggs, oregano, black pepper, and salt. Add the arugula, peppers, cheese, and onion to the slow cooker. Slowly add the egg mixture over the vegetables until they are mostly submerged. Set your slow cooker on low heat for 2-3 hours.

Strawberry Oatmeal Smoothie
1 serving total, 234 calories per serving, 4 grams fat, 45 grams carbs, 7.9 grams protein

Ingredients:
a handful of fresh or frozen strawberries
1 banana
.5 cup rolled oats
.5 cup milk
a pinch of cinnamon

Directions:
In a blender, combine all the ingredients and blend until smooth.

Savory Oatmeal Breakfast
2 servings total, 326 calories per serving, 17 grams fat, 15 grams protein, 30 grams carbs

Ingredients:
.25 cup fresh basil, chopped
.5 cup oats
1 tomato, diced
2 eggs
2 tbsp cheese (Feta), crumbled
2 tbsp milk
pinch of salt and black pepper

Directions:
First pre-set your oven to 375 degrees F. In a skillet, add some water and let it boil before adding the oats. Stir until they become tender according to your package instructions. Mix together the basil, oatmeal, and tomatoes and add salt and pepper to taste. Whisk your milk and eggs together in a separate bowl before combining the two mixtures then dividing the mixture into 2 small baking dishes or ramekins. Top with the feta cheese. You want to bake until your egg mixture is set for 20 to 25 minutes.

Islands Green Smoothie
1 serving total, 223 calories per serving, 3 grams fat, 3 grams protein, 50 grams carbs

Ingredients:
1 cup baby spinach
.75 cup almond milk
.5 cup fresh or frozen pineapple chunks

1 frozen or fresh banana

Directions: In a blender, combine all your ingredients and blend until smooth.

Mediterranean Breakfast Toast
1 serving, 371 calories per serving, 5.8 grams fat, 16 grams protein, 13 grams fiber, 80 grams carbs

Ingredients:
1 slice of whole wheat bread
2 slices of tomato
pinch of salt and black pepper
2 tbsp hummus
3-4 slices cucumber

Directions:
Toast your bread and spread the hummus. Add your tomatoes and cucumber and lightly season with a squeeze of lemon juice as well as black pepper and salt.

Chapter 8: Mediterranean Diet Lunch Recipes

Lentil, Shrimp and Bean Salad
4 servings total, 347 calories per serving, 8.9 grams fat, 38 grams carbs, 19.5 grams protein

Ingredients:
.5 bell pepper, chopped
5-7 mint leaves, chopped
2 tspn capers
2 tspn garlic, minced
1 can brown lentils ~15 oz
7 oz cooked shrimp
2 tbsp white wine vinegar
1 can white beans ~15 oz
salt and black pepper to taste
2 tbsp extra virgin olive oil
.5 tspn ground cumin
.5 tspn paprika

Directions:
Mix together the shrimp, pepper, capers, white beans, lentils, mint, and minced garlic. Season with the spices and add the white wine vinegar and olive oil as a dressing. Stir so everything is well designed. This is a great meal with a slice of your favorite whole wheat pita bread.

Mediterranean Tomato Salad with Fresh Herbs
3 servings total, 125 calories per serving, 9.7 grams fat, 8 grams carbs, 1.6 grams protein

Ingredients:
salt and black pepper
2 oz cheese (Feta), crumbled

.5 cup fresh dill, chopped
4-6 fresh mint leaves, chopped
.5 tspn paprika
3 tspn olive oil
2 tspn garlic, minced
2 tspn lemon juice
2 tspn white wine vinegar
.5 cup onion, finely diced
5 tomatoes, diced

Directions:
Combine the onions, tomatoes, herbs and the garlic in a bowl, then season with your spices (salt, black pepper, paprika). To create your dressing, in a separate bowl first mix together the olive oil, vinegar, and lemon juice. Taste for salt. Top with feta cheese.

Shrimp Avocado Garlic Bread
5 servings total, 222 calories per serving, 7.9 grams fat, 24 grams carbs, 2 grams fiber, 13 grams protein

Ingredients:
.5 loaf of sourdough bread cut into 5 slices about 1" thick
1 tspn of olive oil to drizzle or olive oil spray

Garlic Shrimp:
2 tspn lemon juice
.5 pound peeled shrimp
.5 tspn salt
.5 tspn paprika
1 tspn minced garlic
.5 bunch fresh parsley, chopped
.5 tspn black pepper
2 tspn olive oil

Avocado Salad:
.5 avocado, peeled
1 small tomato, cubed
a pinch of salt
1 tablespoon lemon juice

Directions:
On a lined baking sheet, arrange your bread and brush on a little bit of olive oil. Broil until lightly golden brown. Then prepare the rest of your ingredients. To cook the garlic shrimp, mix the garlic, lemon juice and shrimp in a bowl and add your seasonings (paprika, salt, black pepper). Add some olive oil to a pan and fry your shrimp. Set aside and garnish with parsley. To make your avocado salad, mix all your ingredients and add the shrimp. Add your now combined shrimp and avocado to the bread you toasted.

Quinoa Veggie Wrap
2 servings total, 328 calories per serving, 9grams fat, 49 grams carbs, 13 grams protein

Ingredients:
2 whole wheat tortillas
.25 cup hummus
1 tablespoon sun-dried tomatoes
1 cup fresh baby spinach
.5 cup quinoa, uncooked
.25 cup carrots, chopped

Directions:
First, cook your quinoa but cooking it in 1.5 cups of water or broth. Let it boil then simmer until it is cooked then turn off the heat. In the 2 tortilla bread, divide your baby spinach, hummus, carrots, tomatoes, and quinoa. Wrap like a burrito. You can pan fry to add some color or grill on a panini press if you prefer.

Green Bowl with Chicken and Herbs
1 serving total, 442 calories per serving, 19 grams fat, 31 grams protein, 44 grams carbs

Ingredients:
1 cup broccoli florets
2 cups fresh baby spinach
pinch of salt and black pepper
.5 cup onion, finely minced
1 cup asparagus, chopped
juice and zest of 1 lemon
3 tspn olive oil
.25 avocado, pitted and cubed
3-4 oz leftover cooked chicken, shredded
.25 cup fresh herbs, minced

Directions:
Add some of the olive oil to a skillet to sauté the onions as you lightly season with salt. Cook until translucent then add your other veggies – the broccoli and asparagus and cook until the spinach has wilted. Season with the lemon juice and zest and then cook the chicken. Remove from heat and garnish with the avocado and fresh herbs. Add the last tablespoon of olive oil as a dressing.

Chicken Noodle Soup
4 servings total, 162 calories per serving, 7 grams fat, 13 grams protein, 11.8 grams carbs

Ingredients:
1 can vegetable broth ~15 oz can
3 cans chicken broth ~15 oz can
.5 pound cooked chicken breast shredded

.5 onion, chopped
.5 cup celery, chopped
1.5 cup whole wheat pasta
.75 cup carrots, chopped
1 tablespoon olive oil
1 tspn dried oregano
1 tspn dried basil
.5 tspn black pepper

Directions:
In a large pot, add the olive oil then and add the vegetables: celery, carrots, onion and sauté until it becomes tender. Add your chicken and vegetable broths, and the cooked chicken, along with the noodles, and spices. To cook the soup, let it boil for a bit then simmer on low.

Black Bean and Couscous Salad
2 servings total, 255 calories per serving, 7.3 grams fat, 42 grams carbs, 10 grams protein

Ingredients:
.25 cup chicken broth
.25 cup couscous
1 tspn lemon juice
.5 tspn red wine vinegar
1 tablespoon olive oil
.25 cup corn kernels
.5 bell pepper, diced
2 green onions, chopped
A handful of fresh parsley, roughly chopped
1 can black beans ~15 oz

Directions:
Let the chicken broth boil in a pan. Cook the couscous in the broth according to the instructions then remove to a separate dish once done. Mix together the vinegar, olive oil, and lemon juice. Add your parsley, corn, beans, green onions, and bell pepper. Break up the couscous and mix it with the vegetables.

Whole Wheat Tuna Sandwich
2 servings total, 321 calories per serving, 28 grams protein, 11 grams fat, 28 grams carbs

Ingredients:
1 can tuna, drained ~12 oz
4 slices whole wheat bread
pinch of salt and black pepper
1 tablespoon sun-dried tomatoes, chopped
2 oz Parmesan cheese, grated
.25 cucumber, sliced
2 tspn lemon juice

Directions:
Mix your tuna, sun-dried tomatoes, and lemon juice and season with salt and black pepper. Next, toast your slices before adding your tuna mixture to 2 slices. Add the cucumber slices and cheese. You can heat further in a skillet or panini press if you prefer.

Lentil Burrito Wraps
3 servings total, 305 calories per serving, 44 grams carbs, 10 grams protein, 10 grams fat

Ingredients:
2 tspn garlic, minced
.5 cup dried lentils

.5 cup onion, minced
1 tomato, diced
1 tspn taco seasoning or garam masala seasoning
3 whole wheat tortillas
.25 cup chicken broth or veggie broth
1 tablespoon olive oil
salt and black pepper to taste
a handful of fresh parsley, chopped

Directions:
Sauté your onion and garlic in a skillet in olive oil. Add your lentils and season with pepper and salt, and mix until well combined. Bring the broth to a boil to finish cooking the lentils. Once cooked, you can mash them to become soft. Add the chopped tomatoes. Heat your tortillas and add the lentil mixture and garnish with fresh parsley and a squeeze of lemon juice.

Individual Greek Pita Pizzas
2 servings total, 725 calories per serving, 20 grams protein, 39 grams carbs, 56 grams fat

Ingredients:
2 tbsp lemon juice
2 pita bread rounds
.25 cup mozzarella cheese
3 tspn olive oil
2 cups fresh spinach
.25 cup grape tomatoes, halved
6-8 olives, sliced
.25 tspn dried oregano, dried basil, and garlic powder

Directions:
Set your oven to 375 degrees F. Mix the herbs, garlic powder, and lemon juice and olive oil into the mixture. Arrange your pita bread and brush with

olive oil. You should still have half the mixture left over, you only should use a few drops. In another bowl, combine the olives, spinach, and tomatoes. Arrange the veggies on the tray and drizzle them with the leftover olive oil Sprinkle your pizza with mozzarella cheese. You can bake anywhere from 6 to 8 minutes until your cheese turns brown

Mediterranean Bean Salad
4 servings total, 197 calories per serving, 8 grams fat, 25 grams carbs, 7 grams protein

Ingredients:
2 tbsp olive oil
.5 can of red kidney beans ~15 ounce can
.5 can garbanzo beans
.5 can cannellini beans
salt and black pepper to taste
1 tspn garlic, minced
3 tspn lemon juice
.5 onion, minced
1 tablespoon fresh parsley, minced

Directions:
Mix together all your ingredients. You can season with some salt and pepper and ensure everything is well combined.

Chapter 9: Mediterranean Diet Dinner Recipes

Mediterranean Veggie Chicken
3 servings total, 291 calories per serving, 6 grams fat, 12.7 grams carbs, 3.8 grams fiber, 45 grams protein

Ingredients:
1 tspn of Himalayan salt or regular salt, black pepper, paprika
3 green onions, chopped
2 large boneless skinless chicken breasts
2-3 tomatoes, diced
2 small jalapeno peppers, de-seeded and thinly sliced
2 tbsp lemon juice
1 bell pepper, chopped

Directions:
Mix your lemon juice with spices and use the mixture to season your chicken breasts. On a lined baking tray, place your chicken breasts and chopped vegetables. Bake for 30 to 35 minutes at 450 degrees F covered with foil to trap the moisture. Once cooked, you can broil it for a few minutes to add more color to your chicken.

Crab Cakes
4 servings total, 218 calories per serving, 14 grams protein, 15 grams fat, 6 grams carbs

Ingredients:
8 oz crabmeat
.5 cup whole grain bread crumbs
1 egg
4 tspn lemon juice
.5 tspn salt
.5 tspn dried oregano herbs

3-4 fresh basil leaves, finely chopped
.5 tspn chili flakes
.5 tspn black pepper
2 tbsp olive oil
.25 cup onion, finely minced

Directions:
Mix together the egg, oregano, basil, onion, lemon juice, and the crabmeat. Gently stir and gradually incorporate the bread crumbs so the mixture becomes to the desired texture. Form the mixture into 4 evenly sized round patties using the palms of your hands. (If your hands become sticky from the mixture, apply a few drops of olive oil to help you handle the meat.) In a small pan, add your olive oil and fry your crab cakes on both sides until they are cooked through and golden in color. Now that you have them made, you can eat them with quinoa, rice, or add to a healthy salad for a delicious source of protein.

Lentil Soup
3 servings total, 347 calories per serving, 49 grams carbs, 18 grams protein, 10 grams fat

Ingredients:
.5 onion, chopped
.5 cup carrots, chopped
3 tbsp olive oil
1 bay leaf
1 tablespoon vinegar
.5 cup celery, chopped
2 tspn garlic, minced
.5 tspn dried oregano
1 cup dry lentils
.5 tspn salt
2 tomatoes, chopped

4 cups of water
.5 tspn dried basil
.5 cup spinach, chopped
.5 tspn black pepper

Directions:
Add the olive oil to a large pot and sauté your celery, onions, and carrots until the veggies become soft. Next, add your dried herbs, the bay leaf, and the minced garlic and stir until everything is well combined with the herbs. Then add the lentils, water, and tomatoes. In order to cook your lentils, raise the heat then let the mixture simmer for 15 to 20 minutes. Stir in your spinach and when it wilts, you can turn off the heat and add your seasoning (vinegar, salt, and black pepper.

Risotto with Mushrooms
3 servings total, 405 calories per serving, 12 grams fat, 61 grams carbs, 20 grams protein

Ingredients:
.5 pound farro, rinsed
2 tbsp olive oil
.5 cup frozen peas
salt and black pepper to taste
.25 cup fresh basil, chopped
2 oz Parmesan cheese, grated
3-4 cups hot water
10-12 fresh mushrooms, sliced
4 cloves garlic, minced

Directions:
In a Dutch oven or a large pot, heat your olive oil and sauté the minced garlic and the sliced mushrooms. Season with some salt until your garlic turns light brown and fragrant. Add the farro to the pan and cook in boiling water. Let

the mixture boil, then simmer, so it cooks according to its package timing instructions. Add the peas and cook until the farro is tender. If it's not cooked all the way, you can add additional water. Once the water has evaporated and the farro has cooked, top with the basil and Parmesan cheese and season with salt and black pepper.

Zoodles with Avocado and Mango Sauce
2 servings total, 472 calories per serving, 26 grams fat, 10 grams protein, 61 grams carbs

Ingredients:
1 mango, peeled and chopped or 1 cup frozen mango cubes
1 1" piece of ginger
.25 cup full fat coconut milk
salt, black pepper, and chili flakes to taste
2 zucchinis spiralized into noodles (or pre-packaged)
2 tbsp tamari sauce
1 avocado, peeled and pitted
6-8 mint leaves

Directions:
In a blender, blend the mint leaves, ginger, coconut milk, tamari sauce, mango, avocado, and chili flakes. Blend until smooth and creamy and season with salt and black pepper. Combine your sauce and zucchini noodles and stir until everything is well combined.

Steamed Mussels
4 servings total, 419 calories per serving, 24 grams protein, 27 grams carbs, 14 grams fat

Ingredients:
3 tbsp olive oil
1 jalapeno or chili pepper, minced

4 fresh tomatoes, chopped
8-10 basil leaves, chopped
3-4 cups low sodium vegetable broth
1 cup onion, chopped
3 tspn garlic, minced
.5 cup light or heavy cream
3 pounds fresh mussels
1 tablespoon corn starch
2 cups white wine
salt and black pepper to taste

Directions:
Add your olive oil and lightly sauté the garlic and onions in a pan, until golden brown. Next, add in the pepper, tomatoes, basil, white wine, and the vegetable broth. Make the corn starch slurry by adding the corn starch in a few tbsp of the cream and stirring well to make a cloudy, gray mixture. Then add the corn starch mixture and the cream into the pot. Keep at a boil and let it cook and get thick before adding the mussels. Stir until everything is well combined and let it cook for 8 to 10 minutes until the shells have opened.

One Skillet Mediterranean Chicken with Tomatoes
4 servings total, 137 calories per serving, 7 grams fat, 11.8 grams carbs, 9.7 grams protein

Ingredients:
.5 cup dry white wine
2 tspn garlic, minced
1 tablespoon lemon juice
4 boneless skinless chicken breasts
1 cup onion, chopped
2 tomatoes, diced
1 tablespoon dried oregano

.5 cup low sodium chicken broth
.25 cup olives, sliced
.5 tspn salt
.25 cup fresh parsley, chopped
3 tbsp olive oil
.5 tspn black pepper

Directions:
Make sure your chicken breasts are dry and cut some slits in them to ensure they become well seasoned. Add some minced garlic into the cuts and then season the breasts with half of the dried oregano, some of the olive oil, salt, and black pepper. Add the rest of the olive oil to a skillet. Cook the chicken until both sides are browned. Add the white wine and let it reduce halfway before adding the chicken broth and lemon juice. Add the rest of the oregano and stir to infuse with the spice. Cover the pan and let the chicken cook, turning over once or twice to ensure both sides are cooked evenly. Uncover and add your vegetables and cook until tender. Serve with fresh parsley as a garnish.

One Pan Mediterranean Chicken Orzo
4 servings total, 482 calories per serving, 23 grams fat, 33 grams carbs, 33 grams protein, 2 grams fiber

Ingredients:
.5 tspn salt, black pepper
1 tablespoon fresh herbs of your choice, chopped
1 cup whole wheat orzo
1 pound chicken breasts
4 oz fresh spinach
10-12 cherry tomatoes, halved
.5 cup olives, sliced
.25 cup white wine
3 tbsp olive oil
1 tspn minced garlic

.5 tspn chili flakes
.5 tspn dried herbs of your choice

Directions:
Season your chicken with salt and pepper. Pan fry your chicken in half the olive oil until is cooked through and light brown on both sides. Once cooked, set aside. In another small pot, set some water to boil and cook the whole wheat orzo by following the package instructions. In the chicken pan, add the rest of the olive oil and add the minced garlic, cherry tomatoes, and white wine. Cook until the wine begins to reduce. Once the tomatoes become soft, add the cooked orzo, spinach, spices, and olives, and fresh herbs as a garnish. Remove from heat and serve with the cooked chicken.

Grilled Fish with Avocado Dressing
4 servings total, 661 calories per serving, 30 grams fat, 49 grams carbs, 57 grams protein

Ingredients:
Dressing:
pinch of salt and black pepper
1 cup yogurt
1 avocado, pitted
2 cloves garlic, mashed
3 tspn lemon juice

Salad:
6 cups romaine lettuce, torn
1 can black beans ~15 oz
.5 tspn salt & black pepper
1 cup shredded cheese of your choice
4 halibut fish fillets ~6 oz each
1 cup diced tomatoes
1.5 cups whole wheat tortilla strips or pieces torn

juice of 1 lime or lemon

Directions:
Make your dressing by combining the avocado, yogurt, garlic, and lemon juice into a blender. Blend until creamy and season with salt and pepper. Pre-heat your grill and season your fish fillets with salt, pepper, and lemon or lime juice. Grill until the fish is cooked and then prepare the salad by layering the lettuce, beans, cheese, tortilla, tomatoes in a plate. Add the fish and then the dressing.

Mediterranean Pasta Salad
2 servings total, 344 calories per serving, 14 grams fat, 44 grams carbs, 10 grams protein

Ingredients:
1 tspn lemon juice
salt, chili flakes, black pepper to taste
.25 cup cheese (Feta), crumbled
.25 cup black olives, sliced
1 tspn minced garlic
.5 bell pepper, diced
1 cup whole wheat spiral pasta
2 tbsp olive oil
.5 tomato, diced

Directions:
Combine the olive oil, lemon juice, and minced garlic in a bowl to make your salad dressing. In a large pot, cook your pasta by following the package instructions. Once it is cooked, add to a large mixing bowl so you can combine your other ingredients. Add the olives, feta cheese, tomato, and bell pepper. Dress the salad with your garlic, lemon juice, and olive oil mixture. You can season with chili flakes, salt, and black pepper seasoning and combine well.

Quick Fish Tacos
4 servings total, 413 calories per serving, 16 grams fat, 30 grams protein, 39 grams carbs

Ingredients:
.25 cup reduced sour cream
1.5 cups shredded red cabbage
.25 cup green onions, chopped
.5 tspn salt
.5 tspn black pepper
2 tbsp olive oil
.5 pound tilapia fillets cut into strips
.25 cup fresh parsley, chopped
4 whole wheat tortillas
2 tbsp olive oil
1 jalapeno pepper, thinly sliced

Directions:
Season your tilapia strips with salt and black pepper. In a separate bowl, combine the lemon juice and sour cream. You can season with black pepper and salt. You want to keep half the mixture aside to use later. In a large bowl, combine the jalapeno, cabbage, green onions, and half the sour cream mixture. Pan fry your fish on both sides in the olive oil until the fillets are flaky and golden. Heat the tortillas and add the cabbage slaw, fish, fresh cilantro, and the reserved sour cream mixture.

Grilled Lobster Tails
2 servings total, 740 calories per serving, 45 grams protein, 4 grams carbs, 60 grams fat

Ingredients:
2 lobster tails ~10 oz each
1 tablespoon lemon juice

1 tspn salt
.5 tspn garlic powder
.25 cup olive oil
.5 tspn cumin powder
2 cloves garlic, minced
1 tspn paprika

Directions:
Pre-heat your grill to medium heat. Make your marinade by combining the garlic, lemon juice, and olive oil, and additional spices. Be sure everything is well combined. Use a knife or lobster utensil to split your lobster tails lengthwise. Brush the lobster flesh with the marinade. You want to grill them with the flesh side down on the heat. Keep your cook time around 7 to 10 minutes because the flesh is very tender. Be sure to turn it over once and re-applying the marinade. Remove from heat once done.

Mediterranean Shrimp Skillet
4 servings total, 421 calories per serving, 7 grams fat, 47 grams carbs, 39 grams protein

Ingredients:
8 oz angel hair pasta
salt and black pepper to taste
1 pound shrimp, peeled
2 tspn garlic, minced
2 tbsp olive oil
3 oz cheese (Feta), crumbled
2 tbsp lemon juice
2 tspn corn starch powder
2.5 cups fresh spinach, torn
1 cup chicken broth, low sodium
1 tspn basil herbs, dried

Directions:

Cook your pasta by following the package instructions. Set aside and then begin to cook your shrimp in a skillet with a little olive oil, minced garlic, and salt and pepper seasoning. Remove from heat once cooked. In the same skillet, you can add half the chicken broth, dried basil herbs, and lemon juice. To make your corn starch "slurry," combine the corn starch with the rest of the chicken broth to make a mixture that is thick and gray in color. Stir into the pan to thicken your mixture as you raise the heat. Return your shrimp to the pan, and cook your spinach until it has become wilted. Then you can return the pasta to the dish and garnish with feta cheese. Turn off heat when the cheese becomes melted.

Conclusion

Thank you for making it to the end of *The Mediterranean Diet for Beginners*. We hope that this book has provided you with the information and answers you are seeking regarding the Mediterranean diet. Our goal was to provide a thorough look at this diet and all the advantages and disadvantages it can bring to your life. As always, when making dietary changes you should consult your physician first to ensure this is a healthy change for you to achieve your goals in regards to your individual health. With the Mediterranean diet, much research has proven it is the most efficient method to lose weight and improve your overall health. How easy it is to follow is another bonus! These benefits tend to outweigh the few negative factors that you can adjust around.

With this book, wanted to provide a detailed look at the Mediterranean lifestyle and exactly what it entails. The more informed you are about this diet and exactly what you should and should not be eating, the greater your chances of success will be! We've shared about the history behind the Mediterranean diet and how the research proves the many multiple health benefits this diet can provide. People who go Mediterranean can lose more weight, lower their risk factors of heart disease, and even preserve your bone mass and muscle mass later in life! By keeping your cells more active and healthy, you can slow down the process of aging that affects all of us over time. There can be a few disadvantages to the Mediterranean diet that people have to adjust to, but with the many health benefits, it's obvious that the good outweighs the bad. Without the need to count calories or weigh your portion sizes, the ease of flexibility this diet provides makes it so appealing to many.

It's important to note that the Mediterranean diet isn't just about diet - it's a lifestyle change. You will be focusing on eating a diet with less red meat and more fresh fruits, vegetables, and seafood, but if you truly want to mimic the lifestyle of the Mediterranean, you have to incorporate physical activity into your routine. The people of this region naturally fit exercise into their daily lives whether it was through walking, swimming, or boating. To gain the same health benefits, you should try and be more active in your life to gain those similar health benefits. Even if you aren't going to the gym, try and make more conscious choices to burn calories and get your body moving. You could take a walk around the block, jog, or bike, or spend some time gardening. Simply making the decision to be more active allows you to expend calories and lose more weight.

To help you succeed, we have included many tips for weight loss and how to implement the Mediterranean diet into your lifestyle long-term. It's important you know exactly what habits and foods you should be incorporating in your routine, like staying hydrated, having a diet full of fiber, and planning a mealtime schedule to avoid excess snacking. The more you are able to sustain a healthy diet, the less likely you will be to reach for the "forbidden" items like sugary snacks, processed foods, soda, or candy. It is important you remind yourself of all the things you can eat on the Mediterranean diet versus what you cannot eat. There are so many varieties of food you can include in your meals like vegetables, whole grains, fish, seafood, beans, and even fruit! Some diets restrict fruit due to their natural sugars and net carbs, but the Mediterranean diet urges you to use fruit to satisfy your sweet tooth! You can even have your glass of your favorite wine if you are a wine drinker, but it's important you speak to your physician to ensure that you can drink alcohol with your individual health needs and condition.

We've included a 14-day sample meal plan to help you get started on your Mediterranean diet with easy and healthy recipes you can meal prep beforehand or make in a short amount of time. Not only that, we provide more than 30 recipes for breakfast, lunch, and dinner, so you aren't at a loss at what Mediterranean-friendly meal to make! With this knowledge, you are able to successfully implement this lifestyle into your busy life and gain all the benefits it can offer!

Finally, if you found this book useful in any way, a review is always appreciated!